# A Reason to Smile

Fixing Broken Confidence with Cosmetic Dentistry

# A Reason to Smile

Fixing Broken Confidence with Cosmetic Dentistry

Blue Ocean Publishing Group

Los Angeles, CA

A Reason to Smile
Fixing Broken Confidence with Cosmetic Dentistry

Published by Blue Ocean Publishing Group 19360 Rinaldi St. Ste. 199
Los Angeles, CA 91326

www.aReasonToSmileBook.com

For permissions contact:
barak@dentometrix.com
ISBN-13: 978-1-947436-00-8
ISBN-10: 1-947436-00-7

Dedication

*This book is dedicated to you, the reader,*
*because by picking up this book,*
*you show you care about your oral health.*

# CONTENTS

# INTRODUCTION

This book discusses the benefits of cosmetic dentistry and so much more. It is a resource for you, the patient and the consumer, so that you can learn more about various cosmetic procedures and what they will do for your overall health and well-being. *A Reason to Smile: Fixing Broken Confidence with Cosmetic Dentistry* will help you understand the complex world of cosmetic dentistry so that you can make informed decisions about your oral treatments.

As a dental patient, you have the right to know what procedures are best for you; the risks and benefits of any dental procedure; the cost of all procedures and if insurance will cover part or all of the expense; and what type of outcome you can reasonably expect from the procedure. Unfortunately, many patients are hesitant to ask questions and even worse, are subjected to high-pressure sales pitches designed only to sell expensive dental work by the doctors they should be able to trust.

This book was created to help you understand all the options you have when faced with choices about your oral care. The experts that have contributed to this book have done so because they want patients to understand these procedures. They also want to allow them to make the right decisions about their own healthcare.

Cosmetic dentistry is not a new practice. Archaeological evidence shows that as early as 700 B.C., dentures were made from ivory and bone. Since then, technological advances through the centuries have increased the popularity of cosmetic dental procedures. Certainly, people throughout the ages have recognized the importance of strong teeth; many cultures have also placed a premium on a beautiful smile. The significance of a healthy, attractive smile has never been more important than it is in today's culture. Because of new technology, particularly made possible by the use of computers, you can have the smile of your dreams, provided that you know which procedures will give you the best outcome.

Today, patients are faced with a vast array of cosmetic dental procedures. In fact, there are so many dental procedures available now that it may be overwhelming to consider all the options. Dentists offer services such as:

- Smile Makeovers
- Crowns
- Teeth Whitening
- Periodontal Treatment
- Veneers
- Dentures
- Bridges
- Implants
- Orthodontics
- Children's Dental Care

Patients of any age, from the very old to the very young, can safely receive most dental treatments. There is even sedation dentistry for those who suffer from extreme anxiety about dental procedures or for those who simply want a more comfortable experience.

In *A Reason to Smile: Fixing Broken Confidence with Cosmetic Dentistry*, 12 leading dentists from around the country educate you, the reader, about subjects related to cosmetic dentistry. Each of these experts is recognized as a successful leader in their various fields. In this book you will have access to their knowledge and insight on the following topics:

- The Importance of an Attractive Smile – Allen Ghorashi, DDS, offers insight into how important it really is to have a beautiful smile (hint: it may be more important than you think!)

- To Do It Right, You Need to Start Early – Yasser E. Sadek, DDS, teaches you how critical it is to take care of children's teeth at an early age, particularly if cosmetic dental work is needed

- Crowns… They're Not Just for Royalty – Alan R. Grodin, DDS, discusses the importance of crowns and fillings in today's cosmetic dentistry landscape

- Fifty Shades of White-- Randall Deaton, DDS, discusses the problem of dull, yellow teeth and how to correct it

- Fixing the Foundation: Your Gums – Bryan P. Kalish, DDS, MS, explains why gum health is the key to overall oral health

- Immediate Makeover with Dental Veneers – Steve Tatevossian, DDS, talks about dental veneers and how they can give instant results in brightening and straightening a smile

- Biting Right Is Biting Tight – Brian C. McDowell, DDS, LVIF, helps you understand why your bite is so critical to your overall health and how to make it perfect so you can enjoy years of healthy teeth and gums

- Let's Get Something Straight: Orthodontics – Ernest McDowell, DMD, and Randy M. Feldman, DDS, MS, explain the facts regarding braces, including both traditional and Invisalign methods

- Consequences of Missing Teeth – Stephen DeLoach, DDS, discusses the health concerns regarding missing teeth and how this problem can be solved

- Filling in The Gaps with Bridges and Dentures – Jacob DeVinney, DDS, talks about the benefits of bridges and dentures, two of the most popular cosmetic dental options

- Replacing Your Teeth with Dental Implants – Scott Frank, DDS, helps you understand how dental implants work and whether they are a good choice for you

- No Fear with Sedation Dentistry – Shital Patel, DDS and Rakesh Patel, DDS, offer honest opinions on sedation dentistry and its benefits.

Finally, feel free to jump from one section to another in the book; you do not have to read the chapters in order. Pick your favorite topic and start learning immediately about the things you need to know to make great decisions about your dental care!

*A Reason to Smile: Fixing Broken Confidence with Cosmetic Dentistry* is your guide to making the right choices for your own oral health. Let our experts help you make the right decisions about your dental care!

# THE IMPORTANCE OF HAVING A GOOD SMILE

How important is it to have a good, attractive smile? Here are just a few facts:

- A recent survey finds that 84% of people consider an attractive smile to be "an important feature"

- Roughly the same number, 85% of people, believe a person's smile is "very or somewhat important" in making a good first impression when meeting people

- 90% of people think that a good smile makes a person more attractive

- The American Academy of Cosmetic Dentistry (AACD) reports a study showing that people with good smiles are perceived as more attractive, more successful, more interesting, and more intelligent

- People with attractive smiles are more likely to be hired, more likely to be promoted, and more likely to receive higher salaries

Cosmetic dentistry has become more and more important in recent years, for two main reasons. One, like it or not, people's appearance and image have become increasingly important in society. Secondly, cosmetic dentistry techniques have advanced significantly in the past decades, making it easier for people to improve the appearance of their smile.

In today's society, having a beautiful smile reflects being a beautiful person. When you first look at a person, the face of the person and their teeth play an important role in how you initially perceive them and feel about them. "Eyes" and "smile" are the two most often mentioned features that people find attractive, and between those two features, I think that a really radiant smile is probably noticed first. The simple fact is that a straighter, whiter smile is a very important feature, one that can dramatically affect your entire life – career, relationships, and most importantly, how you feel about yourself.

All you have to do is look at the covers of fashion magazines. You'll always see a very beautiful smile, with perfectly white teeth. That's because the editors of those magazines understand very well how important a beautiful smile is in making a person look attractive. That's why actors, actresses, and models always take great care of their teeth – because they also know that having a great smile is critical to having people find them attractive. We all want to have that same kind of white, beautiful smile.

In contrast, people with missing, chipped, or darkened teeth are perceived as less attractive, even when the rest of their face and appearance may, overall, be very pleasant. And problems with your smile can create a lot of problems in your life. For example, people with dental problems – missing, broken, or otherwise unattractive teeth – have a habit of covering their mouth when they talk to hide their teeth. If you wear dentures, your teeth are always moving slightly when you talk.

The net effect of conditions like those is that people with dental problems usually come off as perhaps a bit shy, distant, or even unfriendly, simply because they aren't seen smiling. Obviously, this can affect how well you do in situations such as job interviews or meeting people socially. People with significant dental problems actually tend to withdraw from interacting with other people because they're self-conscious about their smile. That tendency to withdraw from interactions, socially or at work, can have severely negative effects on a person's life and happiness.

The truth is that your dental health and the appearance of your teeth can play a huge role in your success in life, both personally and professionally. Here's another statistical fact: Researchers have found that people who smile more often actually tend to live much longer, healthier lives.

*Let me tell you about one patient I had, an accountant in New York City, who had upper dentures, upper false teeth. The dentures were ill-fitting and therefore had a tendency to fall out or to break. Of course, he also had problems with eating – with chewing – and with being embarrassed when his dentures fell out. That affected his work and social life because he was reluctant to go out to eat in restaurants, in public.*

*Because he'd had so many problems with his teeth and with earlier dental work, he was also reluctant to seek any more dental treatment. However, I was eventually able to convince him that*

7

*we could really fix things for him and get his teeth right. Anyway, to make a long story short, we were able to fit him with new, properly fitting dentures and it just made all the difference in the world.*

*When I finished the work, he immediately said that he thought it made him look 20 years younger, just because of the way it improved his bite and the overall appearance of his smile. Afterward, he said a lot of his clients remarked that he looked a lot younger, too. It's funny though – most of them couldn't pinpoint how he'd changed. They'd ask him if he'd gotten a new haircut or something.*

*He told me that he became a lot more outgoing after the work I did, and he was very grateful. When you look at his "before" and "after" photos, you can really see how dramatically you can improve someone's appearance with proper cosmetic dental work.*

## COMMON SMILE PROBLEMS

There are several possible problems with their teeth that may lead people to seek restorative and cosmetic dental treatment.

One of the most common reasons is having missing or broken teeth, cracked teeth, or teeth that have worn down by erosion. Any of these problems can first of all cause a person to experience a lot of pain, and that's often something that motivates them to seek treatment. This kind of problem can cause people to suffer pain or to have problems chewing food, as well as the obvious aesthetic problems.

People are concerned with the appearance of their smile. Problems with the appearance of teeth, especially front teeth, is what a lot of patients come looking for help with. People with missing or damaged teeth often want to have those teeth replaced in a very aesthetically attractive way.

Another common cosmetic problem, one that commonly occurs as people age, is that their teeth may have moved or rotated in their mouth, causing them to have teeth that aren't straight, that aren't properly aligned.

In my office, we do a lot of revisions for patients who may have had orthodontic work done, say, 20 years ago when they were teenagers. Their teeth may have relapsed, becoming rotated or crooked again, and so they come in wanting to get that corrected, which we can do with procedures such as orthodontics or veneers, which are thin layers of material placed over a tooth, covering it.

I think patients today show more concern about having straight teeth, and so we see a lot more adults seeking to have their teeth straightened. I'd say that's one area of cosmetic dentistry that has increased significantly over the past 20 years.

Older, amalgam metal or silver fillings can cause people cosmetic dental problems, too. Over time, those metal fillings can become darkened, and this gives the overall appearance of darkened teeth and a less bright, white smile. This is another cosmetic issue that patients may have, the desire to replace those silver fillings with white composite or porcelain fillings. Sometimes patients may choose to repair an older filling by getting a white, porcelain crown.

There's an issue of how much a tooth can handle from a restorative point of view. Sometimes older, larger fillings are putting a strain on what a tooth can handle, and that can lead to teeth cracking or chipping. In those cases, a Porcelain crown might be the best solution. Porcelain crowns offer the advantage of having no metal, and it's also easy for the dentist to match the shade of the crown to the rest of your teeth so that it seems very natural.

Erosion, which can also eventually lead to teeth becoming chipped or fractured, is another problem that can create cosmetic issues for patients. Erosion can occur gradually just from chewing, or from grinding your teeth. There's also acid erosion that can occur as a result of your diet, gradually eroding away the enamel that protects your teeth.

When that outer shell or enamel gets broken down, the teeth become a bit weaker, and that makes chipping or fracture of the teeth more likely. Your teeth may also just get worn down over time, becoming noticeably shorter. We can correct that cosmetically with treatments such as veneers or crowns, which not only strengthen your teeth to prevent any more breakage but also can do wonders for the cosmetic appearance of your smile.

Something else that is a common cause of cosmetic dental problems – a reason that a lot of people are not aware of – is our changing diet. In addition to coffee and sodas that can cause teeth to become stained and darkened, a lot of the health drinks that are on the market and become very popular, because they're made from dark-colored vegetables, these can also cause staining or discoloration of teeth. These factors have led an increasing number of people to seek more dental help with cleaning and teeth whitening procedures.

Teeth problems can lead to major health problems. There are a lot of studies, such as, showing a correlation between gum, or periodontal, disease and heart disease and diabetes. Your mouth is part of your body, so if you're not taking care of your oral health, then the bacteria that accumulate in the mouth around your gum line can enter your bloodstream and cause severe systemic health problems.

It's very important to take care of your oral health because it, in turn, affects your systemic health.

## DEALING WITH MISSING TEETH

Missing teeth are one of the biggest cosmetic issues that people have, especially when it involves a tooth that's right up front, in your smile area, so to speak. Even if someone has an otherwise really nice smile line and nice, bright white teeth, a missing tooth can make someone look and feel unattractive.

Usually when you're missing teeth, the other teeth in your mouth are moving, shifting, even though you may not feel it or notice it right away. When your teeth shift, that can cause problems with changing your bite. Missing teeth also usually cause problems with chewing your food properly, and that can lead to gastro-intestinal or other systemic health problems.

Missing teeth can also eventually lead to bone loss. When your teeth start shifting because you're missing teeth that originally held bone in place, the bone can gradually erode. Bone loss can become a severe cosmetic issue because it leads to an actual shrinking of the jaw and a resulting sunken appearance in your cheeks and facial skin. This can make a person look much older, like a 45-year-old looking like a 75-year-old.

For all of those reasons, it's very important for patients with missing teeth to seek to get that problem corrected as soon as possible. And just as missing teeth can make you look a lot older, replacing missing teeth can make you look a lot younger.

In addition to the traditional treatments using bridges – artificial teeth that are permanently joined to adjacent teeth - or dentures, one of the most important advances in treating missing teeth is dental implants. If you have multiple missing teeth, dental implants can be a great way to restore those teeth in a really cosmetically appealing way.

Unfortunately, now dental implants often aren't covered by many dental insurance plans. It's important to check with your insurance provider. Fortunately, most dentists are aware of this cost issue and so will work with patients, setting up payment plans and that sort of thing.

## ABOUT COSMETIC DENTISTRY

Cosmetic dentistry is not a bona-fide specialty where you go to dental school and then do a specific residency for cosmetic dentistry. What usually happens is that dentists who aim to get very involved with the field of cosmetic or aesthetic dentistry do so through continuing education, getting ongoing education and learning from other dentists with a lot of experience in cosmetic dentistry. It's a rapidly evolving and changing field, so continuing education is critically important for dentists to learn the latest procedures and to gain experience. The best cosmetic dentists are always learning, always seeking to add to their knowledge and skills.

There are some specific programs that dentists can take to learn how to do cosmetic dentistry. There's an organization, the American Academy of Cosmetic Dentistry, AACD, that is right in the forefront of providing education and training for dentists to learn to do cosmetic dentistry the right way and to achieve a proper level of confidence in their skills and abilities. So one thing patients can do is simply ask about what type of education and qualifications a dentist has earned relative to doing cosmetic dentistry.

In my case, I've been doing dentistry for about 25 years and it's like a continuum, you never stop learning. I'm involved with the Academy of Implant Dentistry that has a lot of cosmetic dentistry components attached to it because we take the approach of treating a patient's whole smile and not just treating one tooth.

It's a never-ending field, so you always have to keep learning. You may learn something today, and then tomorrow something new comes out. That's how it works for me, how I stay on top of the technology and techniques, by constantly getting more education and training.

One of the latest advances in cosmetic dentistry is digital dentistry. We now have the ability to take 3-D images of a patient's face and mouth, including the bone and the soft tissue, the gum, and then combine all of those images with software that enables us to digitally design a beautiful smile that's perfectly suited to a patient's individual face. In the past, a lot of things were more standard issue, "one size fits all", but we're now able to customize and personalize a patient's smile by using a computer.

I just want to stress that since there's no specific educational specialization in cosmetic dentistry in dental school, it's important for patients looking to have cosmetic work done to look at what kind of cosmetic work a dentist has successfully done in the past. Don't be shy about asking your dentist about their level of experience. You can also just look at the way a dental practice presents itself. For example, if a dentist specializes in doing crowns or implants, that will usually be clear from looking at their website, the office set-up and or from talking with them.

A lot of dentists who do a lot of cosmetic work will have "before" and "after" photos of other patients that they can show you. I think looking at photos like that can be a key reason in selecting a dentist for cosmetic work. As they say, a picture is worth a thousand words. Do your research, your homework, and definitely interview the dentist before deciding on having him or her do the work you want done.

## COSMETIC DENTISTRY CHANGING LIVES

Good cosmetic dentistry can really change a person's life.

*I had a case not long ago that really made a lasting impression on me because the patient had so many issues coming in, and then because getting the cosmetic work she wanted made such a huge impact in her overall life.*

*When I first saw this woman, she had a lot of dental issues, including being very apprehensive about having dental work done. She was very self-conscious about her extensive dental problems. She had missing teeth, crooked teeth, loose teeth, and gum issues. Because of her teeth not being in the right place, bite problems, and pain, she often wouldn't eat. When she did eat, she wasn't able to chew her food properly, and that led to her also having nutritional problems.*

*Some people don't realize that dental problems can lead to nutritional problems like that, and if you don't get those dental problems corrected, you can actually be starving yourself.*

*Problems with her teeth had also affected her ability at public speaking, which caused her other problems in her life, including a severe lack of self-confidence. This was very important because public speaking was a large part of her life and work.*

*Anyway, because she had neglected seeking treatment for a long time due to her apprehension about having dental work done, I had a lot of catching up to do. The work that I did involved a number of procedures and took a while to complete. It was kind of like building a house, room-by-room, and very much a labor of love for me because I really wanted to get everything perfectly right for her.*

*I had to try to save the teeth I could save, try to remove the teeth we couldn't save, and get her overall oral health back into good shape. It took a lot of work, but when I had finished, the result was that her smile was totally transformed. She was just amazed at the difference, not just in terms of solving practical problems with eating and with speaking, but also with how it completely transformed the entire appearance of her smile and her face.*

*Her smile was just perfect, perfectly customized for her. You could immediately see what a gigantic boost in self-confidence it gave her. At the end of the treatment she had no pain, she could eat better than before, her confidence went up 100% and it was truly a life-changing experience for her.*

I just want to add that having a brighter, more attractive smile will also help you keep that kind of smile throughout your life. Once you've invested the time and energy to transform the way you look, to get that beautiful smile we all want to have, it usually motivates you to take better care of your smile and overall oral health going forward, in terms of staying on top of things like brushing and flossing and seeing your dentist regularly.

Don't be afraid to seek good cosmetic dental treatment. It really can make a huge difference in your life – in your appearance, your self-confidence, your relationships, and the overall happiness of your life.

# ABOUT ALLEN A. GHORASHI, DDS

Valley Dental Group
RamseyDentists.com

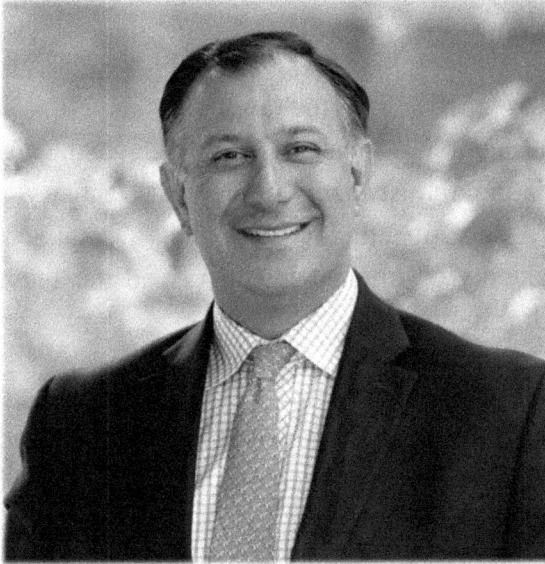

Dr. Allen Ghorashi is a caring and compassionate dentist who focuses his treatment on cosmetic and implant dentistry. He and his team offer commitment to "gentle dentistry" to help patients with their individual needs, communicate effectively and ultimately provide the best results possible.

Dr. Ghorashi attended the University of Oregon where he received an undergraduate degree before transferring to Northwestern University to obtain his doctoral degree in dentistry. He continued his education with residencies in the field of implantology so that he could better understand the needs of his patients. Today, he continues his ongoing education to learn the latest techniques in implant dentistry.

For many years, Dr. Ghorashi has been recognized as a top professional in his field. He has been appointed a fellow of the

International Congress of Oral Implantologists, a worldwide dental implant organization recognized for its high standards of care. He is also an Associate Fellow of American Academy of Implant Dentistry, an honor that he obtained through rigorous peer examination.

Registered to practice in both New Jersey and New York, Dr. Ghorashi's professional memberships include the American Dental Association, the Academy of General Dentistry, the New Jersey Dental Association, the Bergen County Dental Society, the American Academy of Implant Dentistry and the International Congress of Oral Implantologists.

Dr. Ghorashi's passion is comprehensive implant treatment. He begins every case with a focus on the individual needs of his patients, advising the proper procedures for each unique situation. He specializes in complete smile makeovers, veneers, bonding, whitening and aesthetic tooth replacement. In addition, Dr. Ghorashi's group practice provides various dental treatments for his patients, removing the need for them to go to different locations for their dental need.

Dr. Ghorashi and his team are dedicated to providing patients with quality care in a comfortable, state of the art and relaxing environment.

# TO DO IT RIGHT, YOU
# NEED TO START EARLY

Visiting a dentist early and often in childhood can set up a lifetime of healthy results. Genetics dictates physical characteristics from missing teeth to misalignment of the jaw, and cosmetic dentistry plays an important role in making a significant, positive difference as a patient grows. While cosmetic dentistry among adults is on the rise, some procedures can be sidestepped or minimized if parents and dentists partner to adopt an intense focus on early childhood oral hygiene and regular, compassionate and child-centered care.

Every dentist brings a different approach to treating patients, and making the experience pleasant and generally pain-free is the goal. I put a lot of emphasis onto educating the children that come to see me about their dental health. To be effective, I make an extra effort to approach them in a non-threatening manner, which makes them more receptive to the information. When parents bring in their toddlers for their first examination, I examine them in the reception room of my office, looking at their teeth without the big chair and build-up most of us remember from our childhood trips to the dentist. I sit on the floor and play with them.

We have a conversation, and I talk about good brushing and how it is important to clean teeth after every meal. I occasionally read and use my book *A Bug named Yuk* to help create a visual understanding of bacteria in the mouth and the importance of brushing the teeth after meals. During my 20-plus years as a dentist, I have noticed that this approach has benefited my patients over the long-run. Good early oral hygiene prevents worsening problems as children become teenagers and adults.

Dentistry, in general, is the maintenance of healthy teeth, regardless of a patient's age. When it comes to pediatric dentistry, parents play an important role in their child's dental health. The most effective pediatric dentistry focuses directly on the child to encourage his or her buy-in to rid disease-causing bacteria. I educate parents while I talk with their children about how to properly care for baby teeth before adult teeth emerge. This includes discussing the role proper nutrition plays in promoting healthy teeth -- an important factor to avoid traumatic dentist visits that may have a lasting emotional effect on the child.

## SETTING A GOOD FOUNDATION

The foundation for proper dental health starts when teeth are developing as a fetus is forming in the womb. Because of this process, mothers need to support a healthy lifestyle during their pregnancies. This sets the stage for a child's teeth to form fully when they begin to come in. Pediatric teeth, or "baby teeth," start to erupt in the child's mouth at around six months of age, with the lower incisors typically being the first to come in. At this stage, educating a parent on how to care for their child's teeth is crucial. I generally like to bring new mothers into my office, with their child, at the first signs of teeth coming in to offer them tips on caring for their child's teeth.

Many parents ask at what age a child should first visit the dentist for a full examination and cleaning. This is a difficult question to answer because there is a wide range in children's rate of growth and development, and not every child is in the same stage at exactly the same age. In general a child needs to see a dentist by their second birthday, but problems could arise before that and if not addressed promptly they may cause serious complications by the time a dentist sees the patient and diagnoses them. I usually recommend the parents to bring the child in as soon as the baby teeth erupt.

There are situations when a very early visit to the dentist is unavoidable. One mother came to see me with her two-week-old newborn, who was born with lower incisors already protruding through the gums. The teeth were not yet fully formed and set in the bone, but they were causing the infant pain while nursing and were incredibly painful to the mother when she tried to breastfeed. For this reason, I extracted the child's incisors when he was only two weeks old. This isn't a typical case, but I have treated a number of children at a very young age for a variety of reasons. It's never too early to take your child to the dentist; waiting too long may spur complicated problems. I urge parents to bring their children in as soon as it seems necessary, especially if the child seems to have any pain or if they notice problems within the mouth. Seeing a child and treating their teeth as early as possible helps ensure the overall health of a child.

## PROPER ORAL HYGIENE AND BRUSHING AFTER EVERY MEAL

It's important for parents to know how to properly manage their children's oral hygiene, especially because parents are responsible for taking care of their teeth until the children can physically do so themselves. The fine motor skills needed to properly brush teeth don't fully develop until the age of 7 or 8, which means that parents are fully responsible for the care of their children's teeth during those years. Also during those years, parents have to train their children on proper brushing techniques so children can brush their own teeth adequately from the age of 8.

Through talking with parents over the years, I've noticed two common themes among children with chronic dental problems: (1) These parents are not consistent about brushing their children's teeth every day, and (2) These parents let children under age 8 brush their own teeth. Since children thrive on consistency, when parents aren't brushing their children's teeth every day and the oral hygiene regimen is inconsistent, the children are often non-cooperative. And when children younger than 8 years of age are in charge of brushing their own teeth, they just haven't yet developed the fine motor skills necessary for proper manipulation of the toothbrush, so they don't do a good job and end up with tooth decay.

Regardless of age, bacteria develop in the mouth to help break down food that humans consume. Within 30 minutes of eating, food particles left in and around our teeth begin to break down and become acidic. This acid is what starts breaking down the enamel of the teeth, causing teeth to decay and eventually causing pain if not treated properly. This is why it is so important to brush your teeth after every meal.

The American Dental Association (ADA) suggests that teeth be brushed at least twice per day. Based on science, we know that when food is consumed and surrounds the teeth the bacteria in the mouth break down the film of food and make it chemically acidic. Acid, if left for 24 hours in the same spot, breaks down and strips the enamel of calcium. Removing the acidic film once every 12 hours eliminates or at least reduces the possibility of that happening.

However, I recommend to my young patient's parents to brush their children's teeth <u>three times</u> a day because children are constantly eating or snacking. My own daughter finishes dinner and not 10 minutes later asks for a snack. The fact that children graze all day makes their mouth more acidic than adults, which increases the chances for tooth decay. Children also have another factor working against them, with pediatric teeth being structurally weaker than adult teeth -- they are made to be broken down by the adult teeth that are erupting under them. This makes the baby teeth more susceptible to decay, which increases the necessity for more frequent brushing.

## A COMMON MISUNDERSTANDING

One of the mistakes I see parents make most often is a failure to care for their children's' teeth as rigorously as they do their own. Many parents think that because their children's teeth are relatively new, there's no possibility of anything being wrong. Or, that because the baby teeth will fall out and be replaced, that proper care isn't necessary.

Decay is actually much more prevalent in baby teeth because they are softer than adult teeth. The acidity in a child's mouth is also much higher because they eat more often, which is, as mentioned earlier, the cause of decay. But getting cavities or losing teeth is not the only concern. Baby teeth actually play a very important role in speech and self-confidence. Children start developing phonetics like "s" and "v" sounds around ages 4 and 5 and require the use of their front teeth. If baby front teeth are lost prematurely, the children can develop a lisp or a tongue thrust.

Losing teeth early, having discolored or damaged teeth, or having a speech impediment can have negative psychological consequences on a child. Children are brutally honest and will point out others' faults. They may mean no harm, but it can still be devastating for the child and affect his or her self-confidence. Having dental problems and undergoing constant treatment can also cause the child to be fearful of the dentist, especially if the problems become severe and the experience is traumatic. All these issues can be avoided if proper care is given to oral hygiene, accompanied by early and frequent visits to a children's dentist.

## OTHER DENTAL CONDITIONS BEYOND CAVITIES

Barring any serious problems, a child should see the dentist every six months. Because primary teeth are structurally weaker than adult teeth and decay can grow quickly, a cavity in a baby tooth can double in size within six months. It's vital to catch decay early to prevent the need for major reparative work in the future.

There are also other conditions that may cause serious dental problems. Sometimes, developmental problems affecting skeletal development and growth rate of the child necessitate dental procedures to correct alignment. I've seen cases where the upper or lower jaw grows faster than the other and other cases where extended thumb sucking collapsed the upper dental arch. Sinus issues are thought to also contribute to the collapse of the upper arch and may lead to a teeth grinding habit. All these issues need to be diagnosed and treated early to reduce any damage to developing teeth and ultimately the health of the child. In general, I start to watch carefully for developmental issues around the age of four.

Developmental problems are usually resolved and treated using orthodontics. In cases where jaw development and teeth alignment are a concern, it's important for pediatric dentists and orthodontic specialists to work together. Improper alignment affects the wear and tear on the child's teeth and the overall health of the child's mouth.

## THE IMPORTANCE OF AN ELECTRIC TOOTHBRUSH

I often hear from children that they don't like their parents brushing their teeth because it sometimes hurts. This problem is easily fixed by using proper tools and being sensitive to the child's reaction during brushing. We have to remember that a child's mouth is very small and that they are a lot more sensitive than we are. Brushing with a manual toothbrush, especially since children tend not to sit still, can easily lead to jabbing the child's gum or gagging, causing the child to resist. This, in turn, usually causes the parent to push the toothbrush harder into the mouth creating a more uncomfortable experience and parents brushing as quickly as possible to "get it over with."

My recommendation is to use an electric toothbrush (e.g., Sonicare®, Braun®) with a small, soft brush attachment. The electric brush should be used as soon as the first baby molars erupt in the mouth. The brush moves faster than a hand could ever move and does a much better job of cleaning the teeth. The parent can then concentrate on the proper placement of the brush on the surface of the teeth that needs to be cleaned and not make any "brushing" movements. This reduces the chances of hurting the gums and inflicting pain and eliminates resistance from the child. With less resistance, parents are less in a rush and have more time to brush their child's teeth properly.

## THE EVOLUTION OF PEDIATRIC DENTISTRY

Pediatric dentistry has evolved as an industry during the 22 years I have been in this line of work. Technological advances have improved the materials used, but also commonly accepted techniques and practices have changed. In terms of aesthetics, in the past, it was much more acceptable to extract a child's tooth when problems arose. Today, it's far more common to treat teeth before pulling them out, or to find alternative treatments. In the past, amalgam (silver fillings) was one of the most common substances used to repair cavities. The difficulty with amalgam, however, is the size of tooth-reduction required to hold an amalgam restoration in place. Since baby teeth are generally small, sometimes dentists were forced to cause more harm to the tooth than necessary to fill a cavity. Another product that is still used is stainless steel crowns for anterior (front) teeth. Because these crowns are silver in color, they are not pleasing to look at and detract from a child's smile.

With recent advances in composite materials and glass ionomer – a white material used to fill cavities -- there are now an array of dependable tooth-colored compounds that require minimal reduction, and readily adhere to the teeth. There are also esthetically pleasing white-colored crowns for the anterior teeth used in pediatric dentistry, if needed. These advances improve appearance and can help boost children's confidence.

## MY APPROACH

On a personal level, the evolution of my practice has been rather significant. When I started treating children more than two decades ago, the training I had was based on the principal that I should keep the parents away from the child and establish myself as the authority figure to the child. With the parents outside of the treatment room, making me the sole authority figure, I would then make the child comply with my instructions during the dental treatment. This standard treatment method never resonated with me. Instead, I began to develop a new approach to children's dentistry born out of my compassion for children and my empathy toward them based on my own unpleasant dental experiences as a child. My honed approach is what I use today at my practice in Palmdale, California.

After many years of searching, education, and trial and error, today I operate in a completely different way. This new approach revolves around giving all the power back to the child (*Empower the Child*). I take the time to educate every child about dental health. I use the story <u>A Bug Named Yuk</u> to introduce the concept of oral bacteria and the importance of oral hygiene. I then talk to the child and describe the condition of their teeth using age appropriate methods and terminology, before telling them what I would do to fix their dental problem (*Educate & Explain*). The child and I discuss what they can do to stop the "bugs" from coming back and, at that point, I ask their permission to fix their teeth (*Free Choice*).

The time spent in communication directly with the child (and not the parent) builds the child's trust in me. I can tell you that almost always children make the right decision and ask me to fix their cavities. I very rarely deal with upset children in my practice, and I attribute this primarily to the fact that my young patients feel empowered to make their own decision after the trust is built between us.

I urge parents to take part in every appointment because their participation and behavior during the dental treatment is critical to my success. Parents should allow the interaction between the child and myself to be unhindered; when a parent puts their trust in me, the child trusts me. I tell parents to leave their instincts for traditional parenting, where they pass orders down to a child, outside my office. I encourage parents to be in the room with their child at all times, but to be silent observers to ensure children are making their own informed decisions. I have reversed fearful behavior and developed many great dental experiences with previously traumatized children using this method.

Because I've started from a position of trust with the child, they are usually less anxious when we begin. This, astonishingly, has allowed me to rarely use the traditional method of anesthesia when treating cavities in children. I do not use "shots" of anesthetic, and instead only use nitrous oxide gas. The gas helps the child remain in a calm and pain-free state while I perform the treatments they need painlessly. This approach has worked very well in my practice for years with several benefits: the child is no longer anticipating the 'shot,' and they are relieved from that mental trauma. They are also free from the post-operative, uncomfortable numb feeling, which to some children is more uncomfortable and traumatic than the dental treatment. I also eliminated the possibility of the child biting their numb lip and causing injury to themselves after they leave my office. The child can also eat right after the treatment and have a normal rest of their day. This method of treatment has revolutionized my practice and how children perceive dental treatment. It's very rewarding for me to see the children's happy faces when they have a brand new smile.

## WHY I DO WHAT I DO

There's one more story I'd like to share, and it highlights the importance of aesthetics in pediatric dental care. I recently treated a girl, around five years old. In general, children her age are not too self-conscious about how their teeth look. However, this little girl was very embarrassed by the fact that she'd lost her front teeth very early. Sometime around the age of three, a dentist removed her teeth due to bottle rot, which is decay of the teeth usually caused when children go to sleep with a bottle of milk or juice in their mouths. Her mother came in and explained that the loss of the teeth was affecting her daughter in a significant way at school. She told me that her daughter had become less social and had told her mother that she didn't like to smile and didn't want to go to school because she was missing her front teeth. Clearly, this girl's feelings about herself were being negatively affected by not having front teeth. I assumed – based on the strong feelings of this little girl – that she'd probably been picked on by some of her schoolmates.

I treated her by giving her an anterior fixed bridge that I attached to her back baby-molars. I ended up cementing the fake front teeth into place. The impact was instantaneous. She came out of the appointment smiling, and there was a confident glow in her eyes. She later told me she couldn't wait to show off her new smile. Her joy was obvious as I watched her look in the mirror at herself. She hugged me again and again.

I love my job. This is my reward and the reason why I care so much about treating children. I want children to be physically healthy, that's a given. But just as important, I want them to have gained confidence and feel empowered to take care of their teeth without fear being a factor. If I can make a difference through my approach in the lives of the children that walk through my office, then I have achieved my mission.

## ABOUT YASSER E. SADEK, DDS
Palmdale Children's Dental
PalmdaleChildrensDental.com

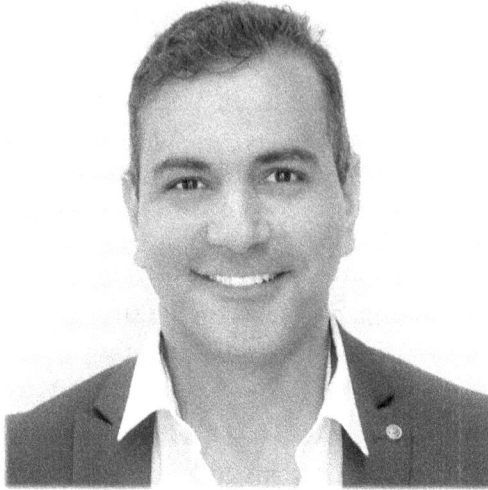

A USC trained dentist, Dr. Sadek has been practicing dentistry in California since 1995. Concerned about the number of children and adults with dental phobia fear, he set about developing an approach to eliminate fear from dentistry. Dr. Sadek's approach focuses on three key features: 1) Assessing the patient's emotional state and elevate/improve it, 2) open communication to empower the patient, and 3) modified dental techniques to minimize discomfort.

Dr. Sadek currently operates a well-established pediatric practice in Palmdale, CA. where his methods are successfully empowering his young patients and helping them receive dental treatment happily. As a published author of, *A Bug Named Yuk* -- a children's book about dental health -- Dr. Sadek has a way of connecting to children and making them feel at ease. Dr. Sadek treats children as smart little people capable of making the right decision once they are educated about dental health. He passionately believes that with age-appropriate communication and changing the children's emotional state from fear to excitement before educating them about their teeth, even the youngest of patients will choose to have their teeth fixed. He gains so much trust with the children that he rarely uses injections/anesthetics and instead only uses nitrous oxide, increasing the safety and comfort of treatment.

Dr. Sadek's dental expertise goes beyond general dentistry and includes endodontics (root canal therapy), implants, and orthodontics. His first private practice in Merced, California was limited to endodontics with patient referrals reaching out from as far south as Bakersfield and north to Sacramento, quickly becoming an authority in the field in the Central Valley. With growing practices and a continuous yearning to excel, Dr. Sadek furthered his training under a local oral surgeon in the surgical placement of implants. A year later, Dr. Sadek further expanded his training by joining an orthodontic practice part-time for a year. There he was able to use his knowledge of implants to accomplish orthodontic treatments that may have been difficult to treat with conventional methods. With the myriad of experiences gained from training and working alongside other experts, Dr. Sadek was able to provide patients with comprehensive in-house dental treatment utilizing implants, endodontics, orthodontics, and cosmetic dentistry.

Dr. Sadek is a member of the American Dental Association, California Dental Association, and American Endodontic Association. He has also served as treasurer, vice president and president of the Yosemite Dental Society. He has always been an active member of the community he serves by donating time and money. He routinely works with the local head start programs, sponsors youth athletic teams and events for the local police department.

ALAN R. GRODIN, DDS

# CROWNS... THEY'RE NOT JUST FOR ROYALTY

White crowns and fillings can be very useful treatments in cosmetic dentistry. Innovations in crowns and fillings have moved them increasingly beyond simply being used as functional restorative dental treatments, making them more effective as cosmetic treatments, too.

## A BRIEF HISTORY OF DENTAL FILLINGS

Fillings have been effectively used as dental treatments for hundreds of years. In the 1800s, fillings were commonly composed of one or another type of metal. Filling materials ranged all the way from mere tin to gold or silver. Whatever the choice of material, the process was essentially the same: the metal was softened so that it could be used to fill in a hole, which we call a cavity in a tooth, to restore the tooth to full function and eliminate pain.

In the late 1800s, dentists began using amalgams. Amalgams are a combination of metals, such as tin, mercury, silver, and copper. The mercury was an important element because it helped to both hold the other metals together and to make them more malleable so that they could easily be shaped and pressed into a tooth, where the amalgam would then harden, restoring the tooth to full function. Amalgams were an important advancement because they both hardened quickly and were strong enough to withstand the forces of chewing.

## ADVANCES IN MODERN DENTISTRY

When I first began practicing dentistry, in the 1980s, amalgams were still the material commonly used for dental fillings. Two events that basically began to occur simultaneously led to a major change in filling restorations. The first was a health concern related to using mercury in fillings. The major concern was actually not for patients, who were at very low risk, but for dentists and dental workers who might be constantly exposed to mercury vapors while doing filling restorations.

In any event, along with some increasing concerns about using mercury, there was also some interest from patients regarding aesthetic and cosmetic factors related to caring for and repairing their teeth. Basically, patients developed more awareness of, and concern about, the appearance of their smile, and so they had a greater desire for dental treatments to not only be functional but also to provide an attractive appearance.

The combination of these two concerns led to the development of composite restorations. Composite restorations are a type of a plastic or an acrylic that is used instead of a metal amalgam. Composites eliminated the need for using mercury or other metals, and also offered dentists the advantage of being able to use white-colored material for fillings that was more cosmetically appealing. In fact, if a dentist puts an effective composite restoration into a tooth, sometimes you won't even notice the restoration because of its cosmetic appearance.

Composite restorations may not be quite as strong or long-lasting as amalgams, but they just look so much better that patients overwhelmingly prefer them. For that reason, I moved completely away from using amalgams in my practice about 15 years ago and went to exclusively using composite restorations for fillings. That's been the overwhelming trend in dentistry over the past 10 to 15 years. I'd guess that there are very few dentists using amalgams for fillings these days.

I don't think there's anything inherently wrong with amalgam fillings, and I don't recommend patients replacing them just because there are now other filling materials available. However, amalgams, like anything else, can break down over the years.

Since amalgams are made of metal, things like wear and temperature changes can occur over time which cause amalgams to either corrode or to pull away from the edges of the tooth, so that they're no longer smoothly fitting in with the tooth. Not only that, but the metal in the tooth can sometimes lead to fractures of the tooth enamel after a period of years.

The bottom line in my practice is that if I see that a patient's tooth is being detrimentally affected because of an old amalgam that's in it, I then recommend replacing the amalgam with a different restoration material such as a composite or porcelain. But I only replace amalgams if there is something wrong with the amalgam or the tooth that the amalgam is in.

I, myself, still have some amalgam fillings that I got when I was a teenager, and those fillings have served me very well. But if they ever needed to be replaced, I would definitely choose to replace them with more cosmetically appealing restoration, either a composite restoration or porcelain. Porcelain – a hard ceramic material - is the other major, modern alternative to amalgams.

## PORCELAIN RESTORATIONS

Porcelain restorations are actually one of my passions. I think porcelain is one of the best options for fillings, or for replacing amalgams. I like the way it looks, I like the way it handles, I like the strength, and I like how it helps to hold the tooth together. When a defective amalgam is removed and the tooth is cleaned up and porcelain is placed in it, it looks like a brand new tooth. It functions very well, and patients seem to love it.

Compared to composite restorations, I just think that porcelain is much stronger, much better for the tooth and for the contacts between the teeth, and for the gingival tissue (the gum tissue). In fact, my hygienists are very strong on telling patients about porcelain restorations because the hygienists are the ones that see the patients every six months and notice how their gums are, and the hygienists tell me that the patients that have porcelain restorations in their mouth seem to have much healthier gum tissue as a result of these beautiful, smooth porcelain restorations.

In my practice, we do a lot of both porcelain inlays and porcelain onlays when a patient needs a restoration or an amalgam filling replaced. A porcelain inlay is a hard porcelain restoration that's manufactured in a lab just like a crown is, and, like doing a crown restoration, the patient wears a little temporary while they're waiting for the inlay to be made in a lab.

The amalgam comes out, the hole in the tooth is smoothed up, shaped, cleaned out, and then two weeks later a porcelain restoration is cemented into the tooth that looks just like the tooth, so aesthetically it's great. A patient with a mouth full of porcelain restorations can actually look like they have no restorations in their mouth, and it allows for beautiful contacts between teeth, which is important for flossing and things like that. Having good porcelain restorations also helps the teeth not to drift, to stay properly in place and aligned.

A porcelain onlay is a restoration that involves one of the cusps, or tips, of a tooth. If, for example, a patient comes in with a partially broken tooth, such as a molar that has four cusps, or corners, one of which is broken, a dentist can create a preparation inside the tooth where an onlay goes into the tooth to replace the missing cusp. It's overlaying the cusp and creating strength for the tooth. You can think of a porcelain onlay as somewhat like a partial crown. Porcelain onlays are used in a number of situations where, in the past, before we had the ability to do these, a dentist would have had to do a crown to repair the tooth.

## INSIDE AND OUTSIDE – FILLINGS AND CROWNS

There are basically two types of restorations that dentists use. A filling is an internal restoration, that is, something that goes within the walls of the tooth. The other type of restoration, a crown, is an external restoration that covers the outside of the tooth.

A dentist uses a crown when the extent of tooth decay is so severe that the breakdown in the structure of the tooth makes the tooth too weak to hold a filling. In that case, the dentist moves to treating the tooth with a crown, a restoration that essentially encapsulates the tooth in a way that retains the form of the tooth and restores the functionality of normal chewing, as well as cosmetically repairing the patient's smile.

## TYPES OF CROWNS

There have been a number of materials used for crowns. Many years ago, crowns, like amalgams, were made out of metals. Gold was used because it was found that gold was a material that was very compatible with the tissues inside the mouth, such as gum tissue and the tongue, and with saliva. The major problems with gold were that gold became increasingly expensive, plus it just wasn't very aesthetically appealing. Therefore, dentists began to develop new materials for crowns that could be used to make white-looking crowns that offered patients a much better cosmetic look.

One of the advances over all-gold or all-metal crowns is a porcelain fused to metal crown, where the crown is composed of metal with a porcelain overlay covering it. The metal makes for a strong restoration and then the porcelain on top of it provides a more aesthetic appearance for the crown. The dentist can choose from a variety of colors for the porcelain, making it easy to match the appearance of the crown to the patient's other teeth.

In addition to the porcelain fused to metal crown, recent technology has enabled us to develop crowns without using any metal. In this category we have zirconia crowns and another type of crown known as an e-max crown. These newer type crowns are all-white crowns that are composed of mostly very strong ceramic materials.

The strength of a crown is a very important factor because of the constant pressures on the tooth from chewing and from things such as temperature changes. Of the newer white crowns, the zirconia crowns are generally considered stronger, while the e-max crowns are generally considered the most cosmetically appealing type of crowns.

There's now a whole range of crown materials that dentists can use to satisfy the individual needs and desires of the patient, and to address different types of situations in the mouth.

A well-fitted crown that's made by a great laboratory can last for decades, or even a lifetime, but unfortunately there's no guarantee of how long a crown may last. A crown might end up getting broken after a couple of years, but whenever I place a crown, I'm hoping for many, many years of service. It's just that there are a huge number of factors that can influence how long a crown lasts – the materials used, the strength of the crown, how well the patient takes care of their teeth, their eating habits, etc. For example, a person chewing ice or grinding their teeth can certainly impact how long a crown lasts. So there's no flat answer to how long a crown will last, but again, a well-made crown ideally lasts many, many years.

## ONE-DAY CROWNS

Another innovation, procedurally, is the one-day crown, where a patient comes in, has their tooth worked on, and gets a crown all in one visit.

Traditionally, getting a crown takes at least two visits. During the first visit, the dentist works on the tooth, preparing it to accept the crown, and then takes an impression of the tooth, which is then sent to a dental laboratory where the crown is made. The dentist places a temporary crown on the tooth for the period, usually a week or two, while the laboratory is making the permanent crown. The patient then comes back and the temporary crown is removed and replaced with the permanent crown.

The technology has now advanced to the point where a crown can be made in the dental office itself, without having to utilize a dental laboratory, thus allowing dentists to prepare the tooth and place a crown all in one visit. Because people are so busy these days, one-day crown visits are becoming increasingly popular. However, personally, I still prefer to have crowns made by trained professionals at a laboratory who specialize in doing that.

The companies that make the systems dentists use to fabricate crowns on their own for same-day service are definitely trying to make those systems as simple and dentist-friendly as possible, but I still think the very best crowns – crowns with the best fit, that are stained correctly and really gorgeous, that give the best look possible for the patient – are made by dental laboratory technicians. As the technology continues to improve, I may change my mind on that, but that's my position at the moment.

A lot of patients aren't aware of how important the laboratory that a dentist uses can be. I always make it a point to explain to my patients that creating a really great crown is an art, and that there are two artists involved – the dentist and the dental laboratory. The dentist is like a sculptor who, in preparing the tooth for a crown restoration, sculpts the tooth into the best form possible to receive the crown, and the dental laboratory's job is then to craft the best possible crown.

If both of those artists – the dentist and the dental lab personnel, both do great artistic work, then you get a perfectly beautiful restoration that will ideally last a long, long time. But it's important for both of those artists to be really good at their respective tasks. If you have a great dentist, but a not-so-great laboratory, or a really great lab but a not-so-great dentist, you're probably not going to get ideal results.

That's why I think it's important for patients, when they're choosing a dentist, and especially if they need a crown restoration, to ask for things like photos of the dentist's previous work or references from other patients. One thing I often tell patients is that if they want to know how good a dentist is, call up a dental laboratory that works with the dentist and ask them. The labs receive the work from the dentist and can often tell from that how good the dentist is.

The laboratory that I've been using for many years now is the Aesthetic Porcelain Studio, located in  California. They make my job much easier because I know that I can rely on them to do great work.

## COST CONSIDERATIONS

The cost for filling restorations, inlays and onlays, and crowns, can vary significantly based on where you live. Getting a crown in Beverly Hills, California is probably always going to cost you more than it would in, say, Raleigh, North Carolina. One reason for the variation is the overhead costs of the dental practice. A dentist in Beverly Hills is probably paying a significantly higher price for their office space.

A lot of dentistry is priced according to the labor and time involved, and also the cost of the materials used. So a composite filling, which is done directly in the office, is going to cost less than an inlay, onlay, or crown that involves work done by a laboratory. In my practice, an inlay, an onlay, and a crown are fairly similar in price.

Overall, I would estimate that an average cost for a crown these days is approximately $1,000. One factor that can influence the price of dental restorations is how much an insurance company will allow a dentist to charge for a specific service. In fact, in many cases the insurance companies essentially dictate the fees.

One problem that patients sometimes run into if, for example, they need multiple crowns, is the annual maximum amount that an insurance company will pay. Filling restorations and crowns are generally always covered services under most dental insurance plans, but the dental insurance might have a maximum annual benefit of $1,500, so if the patient needs more than one crown, then the patient will have to cover a significant part of the total expense themselves. Of course, we work with patients to handle payments, because we realize that sometimes patients can't afford to pay the whole expense at one time.

## WHAT'S IMPORTANT TO KNOW

What I'd like for patients to be aware of is the fact that all of these treatments–composite and porcelain fillings, inlays, onlays, or crowns –if they're done really well, by a good dentist working with a good laboratory, they can do wonders for both the appearance of the patient's smile and for the overall health of their mouth.

If a patient has teeth that are on the verge of breaking, or teeth where a little decay is starting, then it's a very worthwhile investment for them to go ahead and take care of the problem before it gets worse and becomes more difficult and expensive for a dentist to repair.

When I examine a patient who has a situation like that, I'll tell them, "I realize that maybe you're not in pain at the moment, and so maybe it seems like everything's okay right now, but what I see here is that some of your teeth are on the verge of having a problem. It could become a major problem, and before that happens – before it becomes a dental emergency on a Saturday night when there's no one here in the office – it would be a good idea to go ahead and improve the condition of the tooth now so that you can avoid major problems later."

It's just better if we're able to control the health of a patient's mouth and the appearance of their smile rather than waiting for an emergency to occur before we do anything. I've done this long enough to know if, say, a tooth is probably going to break within the next year, so my attitude is why not stop that from happening by going ahead and putting a proper restoration in there. It's definitely a worthwhile investment to take a tooth or teeth that have potential problems and just get them solid again so that potential larger problems don't occur.

That's especially true because of the advances that have taken place in filling and crown restorations that enable dentists to do restorations that are both functional and that can significantly improve the appearance of a patient's smile.

## ABOUT ALAN R. GRODIN, DDS

Flossin' In Clawson Smile Studio

FlossinInClawson.com

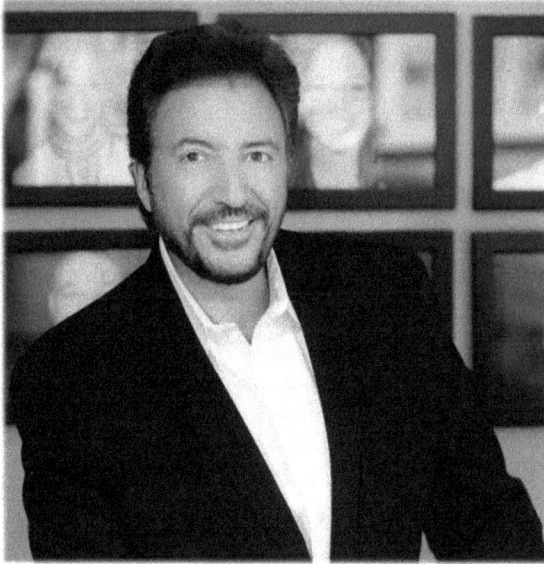

Alan R. Grodin DDS, a Detroit area native, is passionate about improving smiles for his patients. He truly believes that a healthy, beautiful smile helps patients create a better life with more self-confidence. He and his staff work tirelessly to help those who need porcelain veneers and other cosmetic dental treatments.

Dr. Grodin spent his undergraduate years at Michigan State University. In 1982, he graduated from the University of Detroit Dental School as a Doctor of Dental Surgery. He began his work as an associate in the Clawson office, which he purchased in 1987. For more than 33 years, Dr. Grodin has been providing excellent dental care for thousands of patients through his Michigan practice. While his office provides all types of dental service, his passion lies in cosmetic dentistry with a focus on porcelain veneers. Patients travel to Detroit from around the country to avail themselves of his expertise.

Not only does Dr. Grodin provide superior patient service, but he is recognized as a leader in his profession among his colleagues as well. As the "dentist's dentist," he has appeared on the cover of Dental Economics Magazine, one of the nation's most prestigious professional publications. His expertise has helped many other dentists learn the techniques that allow them to provide great smiles for their own patients. He has participated in many workshops, seminars and other professional development opportunities to train dentists in the latest cosmetic procedures.

Dr. Grodin loves to provide smile makeovers, teeth whitening and other techniques for his patients. The goal of Dr. Grodin and his staff is always to help patients achieve the beautiful, healthy smiles they want and to improve their lives with greater self-confidence in their new appearance.

# FIFTY SHADES OF WHITE
## A GUIDE TO TEETH WHITENING

Your smile is one of the first things that people notice about you. It's only natural to want your smile to be as perfect and attractive as possible. Part of a perfect smile is having bright, white teeth.

Teeth whitening has become a very popular cosmetic dentistry treatment and is one of the least expensive. However, despite being generally less expensive than other cosmetic dentistry options, teeth whitening is a cosmetic procedure that can have one of the greatest, most immediate impacts in terms of transforming your smile into an attractive, brightly dazzling facial feature.

*I recall a young lady in her early 20s who came to my practice for help with a dental problem. I could tell that she didn't really care much about her smile, or her overall appearance for that matter. She was just there to get a pressing problem fixed as easily as possible.*

*I asked her if she liked her smile, and her reply was just, "Well, I don't smile." Her response certainly answered my question, even if not directly. The reason she didn't smile was obvious – she had several areas of severe discoloration, as well as several cavities that needed dental restorations.*

*In addition to taking care of the restoration work she needed, I also whitened her teeth. The difference in the way she looked, in the appearance of her smile, was amazing. As she kept coming to my office on a regular basis, everything about her began to change for the better. She began to dress differently; she started wearing makeup again, and she changed her hairstyle from "blah" to "very fashionable" and eye-catching.*

*Eventually, she sent a note telling me that she smiles all the time now. She shared with me that she felt like the teeth whitening procedure had changed her whole life. She told me, in fact, she'd been suffering from severe depression when she first came to see me. But once I restored a bright, beautiful smile to her face, it was like her whole world, her whole life, lit up – like a life that had been completely clouded over by unhappiness was suddenly experiencing the brightest sunny day in the world.*

## THE NEED FOR TEETH WHITENING – THE CAUSES OF TOOTH DISCOLORATION

Unfortunately, it's common for your teeth to become discolored over time. There are several different causes of teeth discoloration or yellowing. One of the main causes of discoloration are the things we drink, such as coffee, tea, and soda.

Other drinks that can stain or discolor your teeth are juices and sports drinks that have high acidity levels. Sports drinks like Gatorade or Powerade are very highly acidic and can wear down your tooth enamel and leave your teeth looking stained.

Interest in teeth whitening has increased significantly compared to what it was 20 or 30 years ago. Dental treatments for teeth whitening are much more common these days. I think there are two major reasons for that.

First, there's just an overall increased interest in cosmetic dentistry. The number of people who are significantly concerned about the appearance of their smile and will do whatever they can to get that flawless Hollywood smile.

Second, our diet has changed in a way that has caused stained or discolored teeth to become a more widespread problem, even for young people, like in their 20s. People are drinking more coffee and soda, also the addition of sports drinks and juices that are often made from dark vegetables can stain our teeth.

Of course, the foods you eat can also contribute to your teeth losing a bright white look and becoming discolored. Some foods, like candy, have a lot of coloring in them, that naturally rubs off on your teeth a bit. I tell my patients, "If something you eat has enough color in it to turn your tongue blue, then you can assume that it will stain your teeth somewhat, too."

Even very healthy foods, including fresh fruits like strawberries, blueberries, cranberries or raspberries, can stain your teeth because they have very high, or very strong, color in them.

Over time, condiments like mustard and ketchup, things that most of us use frequently in our diet, will also cause teeth to stain.

Even if you're not eating or drinking things that are likely to stain your teeth, you're still going to be subject to the natural process of aging. Our teeth gradually tend to become somewhat less white and somewhat more yellow as we age. The enamel on our teeth, the hard, white coating that ideally gives us a nice, bright smile and that also protects our teeth from decay, just naturally wears down over the years.

The rate at which tooth enamel wears down and becomes discolored, and the amount of discoloration, can vary quite significantly from one person to another. Genetics are one factor that determines how quickly or severely you may experience tooth staining. Your lifestyle is another potential factor. Children or teenagers that play a lot of sports consume more of those acidic types of drinks that can eat away at tooth enamel.

There are several other factors that can affect how much discoloration or staining occurs, how fast and how much wearing down of the enamel on your teeth.

Tooth enamel can be gradually worn down by all the things I've already mentioned – coffee, tea, and many of the foods we eat, particularly sugary foods. Tooth enamel can also be gradually worn away by medical conditions such as gastroesophageal reflux disease (GERD), more commonly known as acid reflux disease.

Acid reflux disease is a condition where the sphincter valve that ordinarily prevents stomach acid from backing up into the esophagus – the passageway that carries food from your mouth down to your stomach – malfunctions, allowing stomach acid to rise up into the esophagus or even all the way up into the mouth.

Acid reflux is associated with erosion of dental enamel through a process known as demineralization, which results from a change in acidic levels in the mouth that decreases the oral pH, the relative levels of acidity and alkalinity in the mouth environment. Lower pH numbers indicate higher levels of acidity. Dental enamel consists primarily of a calcium phosphate mineral that is insoluble in an alkaline environment, but that becomes more and more soluble in an acidic environment.

The erosion effects on tooth enamel that result from acid reflux tend to be concentrated on the "maxillary", or upper, teeth. Because research suggests that more than one-third of Americans suffer from heartburn at least once a month and that nearly one-tenth of the population suffers from heartburn as often as once a day, potential enamel erosion and tooth discoloration from acid reflux symptoms are a significant dental health issue.

As tooth enamel gradually wears down or erodes, it exposes the darker part of the tooth that is beneath the enamel, the part called the "dentin". Exposing the dentin makes your teeth appear faded, grayed, discolored or yellow.

## SMOKING AND TOOTH DISCOLORATION

Another factor that can significantly contribute to enamel erosion and the darkening or discoloration of your teeth is smoking, or any other oral use of tobacco. Smoking is a major cause of teeth yellowing. Both the tar and the nicotine contained in tobacco can stain your teeth. Tar is a naturally dark residue from tobacco. Although nicotine itself is colorless, it becomes yellow in color when combined with oxygen molecules.

Tooth enamel, one of the hardest substances in our body, does an outstanding job of protecting our teeth. However, enamel also contains microscopic-size pores where tar and nicotine can collect and build up over time, causing discoloration of your teeth. Fortunately, tar and nicotine stains on your teeth usually affect only the outermost layer of tooth material. They don't usually penetrate beneath the tooth enamel into the dentin.

This is significant in relation to tooth whitening because it means that tobacco stains usually respond well to teeth whitening treatments. The hydrogen peroxide-based gel that is most often used in teeth whitening is highly effective in removing the brown or yellowish stains that come from tobacco. Sometimes, patients who have severely stained teeth as a result of smoking will see dramatically brighter, whiter teeth immediately after getting teeth whitening treatment.

However, I want to note that smoking can cause severe dental problems beyond just cosmetic issues that may be easily treated and repaired. Smoking can lead to serious oral health problems, including periodontal disease, tooth decay, and oral cancer.

A lot of times I have patients come in for teeth whitening treatment after they've just quit smoking. They don't plan to subject their teeth to tobacco stains anymore, so they decide that it's a good time to have their teeth whitened. When I treat patients who are current or former smokers, I always recommend that they get an overall oral health checkup at the same time that they're receiving teeth whitening treatment.

One fact not commonly known is that the side effects of certain medications can also cause tooth discoloration and darkening. Frequently prescribed medications that may cause tooth darkening include antihistamines and high blood pressure medication. It's also been found that very young children who take antibiotics such as tetracycline may experience discoloration much later in life when they begin getting their adult teeth. Chemotherapy has also been known to cause tooth discoloration.

## TEETH WHITENING TREATMENTS — AN OVERVIEW

Patients have a lot of different treatment options to choose from for teeth whitening. In fact, there are so many options that it can sometimes become confusing. I always try to clearly explain to my patients all the various choices available, so that they have all the information they need to make the best choice for themselves.

The most commonly used method of teeth whitening is the custom-fit tray bleaching method. For the most immediate and most dramatic results, patients usually opt for in-office whitening treatments that utilize techniques such as "laser whitening" or "power bleaching". Both of these techniques use hydrogen peroxide as a bleaching agent. They simply utilize different technologies to activate the hydrogen peroxide.

Other whitening treatment methods include using dental whitening strips, over-the-counter or prescription strips.

## WHITENING TOOTHPASTES

Whitening toothpastes are a popular form of over-the-counter whitening therapy. Some whitening toothpastes use the same bleaching agent as more intensive, in-office whitening treatments – hydrogen peroxide. However, the concentration of hydrogen peroxide in whitening toothpastes is usually very low – just around 3% - so it takes a considerable span of time to see any noticeable whitening results. Those results are not going to compare to the results obtained from more professional teeth whitening treatments.

Whitening toothpastes commonly use an abrasive ingredient that works to erase surface stains on teeth by wearing down the very topmost surface of tooth enamel, much in the same way that sandpaper works on the surface of wood. Over-the-counter whitening toothpastes can do a good job of removing surface stains but are not generally as effective as in-office tray bleaching treatments for getting rid of severe discoloration.

Whitening, abrasive toothpastes are usually too abrasive to use all the time. If you use them continually, the abrasives in the toothpaste are going to start to wear away your tooth enamel, so I don't recommend it. Using abrasives too often can also potentially create tooth sensitivity issues or gum problems. But it's fine to use them on an occasional basis to remove surface stains and brighten your teeth.

In essence, abrasive whitening toothpastes are designed to brighten your smile by basically scrubbing, cleaning, and polishing your teeth very well.

For people who want to use abrasive toothpastes, it's important that you know just how abrasive the toothpaste is. This can be checked with a scale known as the Relative Dentin Abrasivity (RDA). In general, the best whitening toothpastes are those with an RDA between 0 and 100. There are a number of websites that list the RDA of virtually all over-the-counter toothpastes.

If a toothpaste has an RDA higher than 100, it should be considered potentially harmful to your teeth and used very sparingly, or infrequently. Regardless of a toothpaste's RDA score, dentists recommend using one that contains fluoride, in order to help strengthen your teeth.

Some people have their own recipes for making abrasive toothpaste using a mix of baking soda and hydrogen peroxide. A lot of people may have grown up using baking soda as toothpaste. It's generally a good abrasive agent but considered too highly abrasive to use every day.

It's very important to be careful with using an abrasive agent because once a part of your tooth enamel is worn away, there's no way to ever get it back. Tooth enamel is not very thick. It's only about one millimeter thick on the front sides of your teeth and about one and a half millimeters thick on the chewing side of your teeth.

## OTHER WAYS OF GETTING WHITER TEETH

One avenue to whiter teeth is to simply start eating healthier. Harder, crunchy foods such as apples or celery actually scrub your teeth as you chew them, and thus will help to remove surface stains.

One of the more recently developed whitening treatments is using whitening rinses. These are mouthwashes that, just like ordinary mouthwashes, reduce plaque and freshen breath, but these specially made rinses also contain hydrogen peroxide or similar additives to whiten your teeth.

Typically, you have to use whitening rinses daily for about three months before you can expect to see noticeable results. Rinses are not going to be as effective as more advanced whitening treatments since they're only "applied" to your teeth for a few seconds at a time. They can help to give your smile a little extra brightness.

Another recent treatment development is dental whitening pens. Whitening pens are simply brush-on applicators that are used to apply a bleaching peroxide compound directly onto teeth. One advantage of this method is that it can be used to treat individual teeth, so it may be a good choice if you just have one or two teeth that are discolored or stained. And it also enables you to avoid the inconvenience of having to wear a bleaching tray.

Regardless of which teeth whitening treatment plan you choose, always talk it over with your dentist. Your dentist can tell you which treatment plans will likely work best for you, and also alert you to plans that won't work or that may actually be dangerous to your teeth and your overall oral health.

## POTENTIAL PROBLEMS OF BUYING TEETH WHITENING KITS ONLINE

There are several companies out there selling teeth whitening treatment kits online. Now, some of those treatment kits work fine, but others are downright dangerous for your teeth, gums, and overall health.

Potential problems include things such as, you might get trays that are improperly fitted so that wearing them could cause serious damage to your gums. Some companies sell whitening kits that use a hydrogen peroxide solution that is stronger than what is considered safe to use.

Believe it or not, some companies even use bleaches that are the same type of bleach that's used to clean swimming pools. Bleach like that is way, way too strong to ever use on your teeth. Using that kind of bleach in your mouth could potentially be extremely harmful to your teeth and gums. You could very easily end up creating more dental problems than you fix.

One study of whitening treatments available on the internet found that two out of every ten people who used a whitening treatment kit that they bought online showed signs of gum damage and/or chemical burns.

The bottom line for choosing a good whitening treatment and making sure that you use it properly, so that you'll get the best possible results while still staying safe, is to always consult with your dentist before deciding on a treatment plan.

## IN-OFFICE WHITENING TREATMENTS

The most reliable studies show that the most effective treatments are in-office whitening treatments that use custom-fit trays that are made in a dental office. With the custom-fit trays whitening technique, the dentist takes an impression of your teeth to create a custom-fitted plastic tray which will hold the bleaching agent used to whiten your teeth.

The plastic trays are custom-made to fit your teeth so that they're comfortable to wear and so that you get full, complete coverage of your teeth with the bleaching solution that goes in the trays.

Dentists sometimes use reservoirs in creating the whitening trays. These are small extra spaces on the front side of teeth being whitened that are designed to hold an extra amount of bleaching agent and thus help to maintain the best possible coverage of your teeth

The whitening trays can also be taken home to wear over your teeth for about 30 minutes to an hour, either once a day or multiple times per day (depending on patient sensitivity and the level of whitening desired), for a period of one to two weeks, after which you will usually see full results.

The dentist places a small amount of whitening gel, which consists of carbamide peroxide, into the custom-fit tray. Carbamide peroxide is used because it easily breaks down into hydrogen peroxide and because it lasts longer than other whitening agents.

The most common treatment process is typically in-office treatments combined with follow-up at-home treatments. On average, in-office visits take no more than 60 to 90 minutes and most patients only require one in-office visit to get their desired effect.

Sometimes a dentist may schedule two office visits: an initial visit, followed by a couple of weeks of at-home treatments, and then a final in-office treatment designed to get the patient's teeth to the exact level of whiteness desired. Using in-office whitening treatments, patients are usually able to have their teeth successfully whitened by somewhere between six and twelve shades.

Teeth whitening treatment is a very individual procedure. Both treatment methods and results can vary significantly from one patient to another. Two major influencing factors are the level of discoloration or staining the patient has, and the end result the patient is looking for in terms of whiteness and brightness. Teeth that are discolored with a yellow or brown shade typically whiten better than those with black or gray hues.

At-home treatments, on average, last about two weeks, with the patient wearing the whitening trays, commonly, for approximately one hour per day. The severity of the patient's stains and their overall level of sensitivity can affect the projected timetable for treatment.

In cases where the patient has extremely discolored teeth but is not overly sensitive, trays can be worn for more than an hour per day to get the teeth to the ideal, desired shade more quickly. On the other hand, patients with extremely sensitive teeth may only be able to wear whitening trays for a total 20 to 30 minutes per day, so they might need close to a month to reach desired results.

In-office whitening treatments offer a couple of significant advantages over purely at-home, do-it-yourself treatments. When performing treatments in their office, dentists take measures to protect the gums and other soft tissue in the mouth from the bleaching agents.

Also, the results of professional, in-office whitening generally last approximately twice as long as the results of at-home whitening treatments – about one full year on average, as compared to only about six months with at-home treatments.

Because the dentist is there during the treatment and able to take necessary precautions, in-office treatments can use a much higher concentration level of peroxide – up to around 40%, as compared to usually only around 5% bleaching agent concentrations for at-home treatments. Therefore, in-office treatments tend to be substantially more effective, and in a shorter period of time, than at-home treatments.

## LIGHT SYSTEMS FOR TEETH WHITENING

A number of dental whitening treatments use light systems to activate the teeth whitening process. Zoom is one of the most popular and widely used in-office light systems. The Zoom system uses an LED light to activate crystals in the Zoom hydrogen peroxide bleaching material. Ordinarily, a Zoom treatment can lighten your teeth up to six to eight shades in just one office visit.

Lumibrite is another very popular system, similar to the Zoom system but using a different kind of light, a plasma arc light that's a different wavelength on the light spectrum, to activate the crystals in its hydrogen peroxide material.

LaserSmile is another light-based option. LaserSmile uses a laser, called a biolase laser, to activate its crystals. The in-office laser whitening technique, which is sometimes called power bleaching, applies a very high concentration of hydrogen peroxide to the teeth, approximately 38%.

For safety, dentists typically use a cheek or lip retractor and a protective covering that's called a paint-on dental dam is to protect soft tissue such as the gums.

One advantage of light-based whitening options is the total treatment time of no more than 40 minutes. Treatment takes less time because the light used amplifies the intensity of the whitening agent's activity.

## KöR Deep Whitening

There are some in-office whitening systems that will use intense light as a bleaching activator, and some instead use a chemical catalyst to activate the crystals in the hydrogen peroxide solution. One well-known whitening treatment that uses this catalyst technique is KöR Deep Whitening, developed by Dr. Rod Kurthy.

KöR Whitening pays close attention to details such as the quality of teeth whitening gels that dentists use. One discovery that Dr. Kurthy made is that refrigeration protects whitening gels against damage or loss of potency resulting from heat during storage and shipping. Following this discovery, KöR Whitening became the first company to maintain refrigeration of teeth whitening gels from the point of manufacture up to the time of delivery to a dentist's office in cold-storage containers.

KöR Deep Whitening is an in-office whitening treatment designed specifically to treat patients with genetic conditions that have led to severe tooth discoloration. Another potential cause of severe discoloration is that is a patient having taken certain kinds of antibiotics, especially Tetracyclineor Doxycycline. Ingesting these antibiotics at a young age can result in a patient's teeth turning noticeably gray.

Ideal whitening results for teeth with this type of discoloration can be obtained when the whitening gels are fully potent, influenced chemically to produce free radicals, and are given a sufficiently long period of time that allows the whitening agent to permeate the microstructure (dentin) of the teeth.

Research shows that traditional whitening gels are usually potently active for only about 25 minutes because of rapid contamination by saliva and the anti-oxidant enzyme peroxidase that is in saliva. To overcome this obstacle, the KöR Deep Whitening system utilizes KöR-Seal™ trays that are specifically designed to seal out fluid that would otherwise contaminate the whitening gel, thus rendering the gel potent for a longer period and ultimately enabling it to produce superior whitening results.

With KöR Deep Whitening, in addition to in-office whitening treatments, patients wear custom-fitted trays, filled with bleaching gel, while they're sleeping, for a period of approximately two weeks.

## MAINTAINING YOUR BRIGHT WHITE TEETH

The level of whiteness and brightness reached with various whitening treatments, and the length of time that the treatment results are visibly maintained, often depends largely on the patient.

Not everyone can have and maintain a super-white smile. For example, some teeth simply don't hold certain pigmentation well.

Some patients have to balance their desire for perfect aesthetics with their desire for comfort.

Regardless of many factors that may affect outcomes, and no matter how bright your smile, in order to keep an attractive smile, it's vitally important to practice good dental maintenance and take proper care of your teeth.

Maintaining a solid oral hygiene regimen that includes brushing, flossing, and using mouthwash is key to making your whitening treatments both effective and long-lasting. It's also important to avoid, as much as possible, foods and beverages that can newly stain your teeth, such as coffee, tea, and some sports drinks.

Some patients may use one of the more advanced, in-office treatments to get the kind of radiant smile that they want, and then after getting that major treatment, they may use touch-up whitening kits with approximately a 10% concentration of hydrogen peroxide to help keep their teeth bright white.

If you do use touch-up treatments, make sure that the touch-up kit does actually use a proper whitening treatment. Some touch-up kits only contain the pigment, titanium dioxide. Such treatments don't actually erase teeth staining. Instead, they just kind of paint your teeth white with the pigment. While that may work well enough as a short-term treatment, the pigment rinses away quickly and does not have the same long-lasting effect as teeth bleaching.

It helps to brighten and whiten your teeth if you just acquire the habit of always brushing your teeth, or at least rinsing thoroughly with water or mouthwash, immediately after consuming food or drinks that are likely to stain your teeth. For example, it helps to brush or rinse right after you finish drinking a cup of coffee.

## COST CONSIDERATIONS

As of 2017, the average national cost of in-office teeth whitening usually ranges somewhere between $450 and $650. For customized, take home trays, patients will generally pay somewhere between $200 and $400. KöR Deep Whitening, typically the most expensive type of whitening treatment, costs significantly more – usually in the range of $900 to $1,100 because the Deep Whitening requires an additional two or three in-office treatment sessions.

Actual costs vary depending on a number of factors, such as what part of the country the patient lives in, and the skill level of the doctor performing the treatment.

There are, of course, over-the-counter whitening trays that are bought and used at home. However, they are not professional grade materials, nor custom-fitted for the patient's teeth. In the long run, I think it's well worth spending a little more for individualized, customized treatment that is going to yield significantly better results.

Because teeth whitening is a cosmetic procedure, it is usually not covered by dental or medical insurance plans.

## OVERCOMING POTENTIAL PROBLEMS WITH TEETH WHITENING

Generally speaking, teeth whitening is a safe treatment procedure for virtually any patient. There are, of course, certain health conditions that might prevent an individual from getting teeth whitening dental treatment. Each individual patient needs to be examined to make sure that their teeth and gums are healthy. This usually entails getting a complete dental exam and having x-rays taken to definitely determine eligibility.

If a patient has significant periodontal problems, gum disease, then they are typically not good candidates for tooth whitening procedures. With patients who have crowns or porcelain veneers, it can be complicated because teeth whitening treatments only affect the color and brightness of natural teeth, not that of artificial dental restorations.

In situations such as those, it might be necessary for the dentist to perform some additional restorative dental treatments like veneers, crowns, or bridges to create a proper situation for all the teeth to be the same shade and brightness.

I don't recommend professional teeth whitening for women who are pregnant. It's better to wait until after your baby is born.

Although the risks have not been pinned down specifically, the peroxide whitening ingredients can potentially be absorbed or ingested during the treatment. There might be possible damage to an unborn child so the wisest course of action is to wait until you're not pregnant.

In the meantime, you can safely combat staining by brushing your teeth with a paste made up of an equal mix of baking soda and strawberries. Try just brushing your teeth with that and letting it sit on your teeth for five minutes before rinsing. Strawberries contain a natural substance that works to break down stains.

## PATIENT ISSUES RELATED TO GETTING TEETH WHITENING TREATMENT

There are several minor problems that patients may experience during or after the whitening procedure. The most common problem I see is sensitivity, usually to extreme heat or cold, as well as to very sweet foods. This sensitivity is never permanent, and it usually occurs only immediately during or immediately after a whitening procedure.

With in-office treatments, sensitivity usually disappears within 24 to 48 hours. One way the dentist can combat sensitivity is by using whitening gels that are less acidic. The dentist can get gels buffered to create higher pH levels.

Personally, I usually recommend using a desensitizer because I've found from my experiences with patients that using a desensitizer immediately after a whitening treatment closes up pores in the enamel, which not only helps with avoiding discomfort but also tends to make the end result last longer.

## A BRIGHTLY SHINING SMILE

At the end of the day, my goal is to provide patients with a healthy, attractive smile that they are excited to share with others. Most of the time, helping a patient to change- to improve - the color and brightness of their smile helps to improve their self-confidence and their overall outlook on life. Getting a really bright, white smile restored is one of those events that you look back on years later and realize how incredibly important it was in your life.

*One patient, a wonderful woman in her early 70s, who struggled throughout her whole life with darker teeth wanted to try the traditional whitening procedure, but that didn't produce ideal results because the staining and discoloration just went too deep.*

*I decided to use the deep-whitening treatment that works all the way through into the dentin. Once the treatment was complete, she saw a before and after comparison of her beautiful smile in the mirror and began to cry.*

*When I saw that she was crying, I thought she might be experiencing some pain, so I asked her if she was all right. And she just smiled through her tears and said, "I'm a lot better than all right. You've managed to do something that I've wanted for years. I'll be forever grateful to you, doc!" Her smile and the joy that it brought her, after so many years of embarrassment and shame, will live with me forever.*

## ASK QUESTIONS

It's important that patients understand the different types of whitening treatments available. I encourage my patients to challenge me with questions. It's important for them to know what they're getting into when they have a whitening procedure done. I urge all of my patients to ask me about every procedure, ingredient, process, cost, and what kind of results that they can, and should, expect. I want nothing but the very best for my patients, and it's impossible to get the right kind of treatment if you can't make an informed decision.

For teeth whitening treatment, I'd want to find a dentist to do the procedure who is really enthusiastic about cosmetic dentistry, someone who's up to date on all the latest treatments. I think that's the kind of dentist that is more likely to deliver you ideal results you want from a cosmetic procedure.

# About Randall Deaton, DDS

Adamsville Family Dentistry

AdamsvilleFamilyDentistry.com

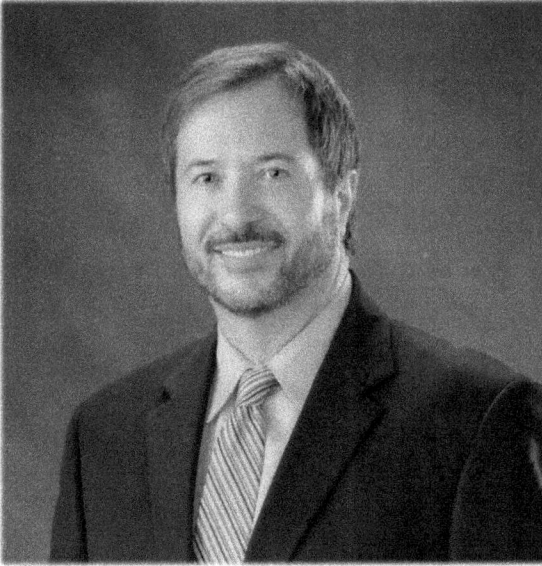

Dr. Randall Deaton is committed to providing his patients with professional and compassionate dental care. He and his staff use the latest technical applications to provide cosmetic, restorative and implant dentistry for patients. They create dazzling smiles that brighten patients' lives and improve self-confidence.

Dr. Deaton earned his degree in biology from the University of Tennessee at Martin, after which he attended the University of Tennessee College of Dentistry, graduating in 1993. Upon graduation, Dr. Deaton began working with patients to provide the best possible care, focusing his practice on cosmetic and restorative dentistry practices. He maintains his skills by attending regular professional development courses, where his expertise and leadership are recognized by his peers. He is a member of the Spear Faculty Club, an organization of dentists who have committed to clinical learning for a lifetime in order to study the latest advancements in all fields of dentistry.

As a leading practitioner in his field, Dr. Deaton also maintains membership in several professional organizations. He is a member of the American Dental Association, the Tennessee Dental Association, the American Orthodontics Society, and the Academy of General Dentistry.

A resident of Adamsville, Dr. Deaton is also active in the community. He is a member of the Adamsville Lions Club and is the liaison to the Retired and Senior Volunteer Program or RSVP. Dr. Deaton is also a member of the band "Riverstone." He can often be found making great country/rock music along with his friends to benefit charities.

Dr. Deaton and his staff welcome patients who are ready to take the next step in creating a new appearance that will enrich their lives. Offering the latest in smile makeover and cosmetic practices such as dental implants, as well as full orthodontic services, Dr. Deaton can help anyone attain a beautiful smile.

# FIXING THE FOUNDATION: YOUR GUMS

All patients should understand the relationship between their teeth and gums by thinking of a photograph in a frame. The teeth are the center point of a photo while the gums provide the support. If the framework is out of line or damaged, then the photo in the center will not appear as beautiful as it would if the border were in perfect working order and alignment.

## ISSUES WITH GUMS AND TEETH

All patients, even those not concerned with cosmetic dentistry, should brush and floss their teeth and gums daily to prevent gum and tooth diseases. In addition to maintaining good oral hygiene, patients should also receive a dental checkup and cleaning every six months. For patients interested in cosmetic dentistry, good oral hygiene and routine dental visits are crucial. With cosmetic dentistry, the first step is to determine whether or not the gums are healthy.

If your gums look red, swollen, inflamed, and bleeding, those are warning signs of an infection. If your gums are infected, then your dentist has to take care of that issue before proceeding to cosmetic dentistry. Again, think of the gums and the underlying bone as the foundation for your teeth. It is critical to make sure that supporting base is solid first, and then the dentist can build on that strong framework to achieve the goal of making your teeth and smile as esthetically beautiful as possible.

Depending on the nature of the inflammation or infection, there are surgical and non-surgical treatments that may be used to correct the problem.

Besides the physical appearance of the gums, it is also important to look at the height of your teeth in relation to your gums – the proportion between your gums and the teeth. If your teeth appear short, this may be because gum tissue is covering part of the bottom portion of the teeth so that they are not visible. This can happen in young adults – men and women in their teens, twenties, or thirties – if their gums have not migrated to their proper final location. The gums have stopped short of settling into their appropriate location, and this can leave part of your adult teeth hidden under your gums.

Your teeth may naturally appear a little bit "short" when you are a child and teenager, but by the time you are a full-grown adult, your gums should have finished migrating to their appropriate position in your mouth. But many times – especially in the esthetic zone – the gums stop migrating too soon, which can give you short-looking teeth.

As you age, the opposite problem can occur – your teeth may appear unnaturally long. That is where the expression "long in the tooth" comes from – which means a person looks old. If your gums have migrated past the point where they are supposed to be, it is commonly referred to as receding gums.

Receding gums cause the "long in the tooth" appearance. Gum recession may occur gradually or rapidly. Many people that show a lot of teeth when they smile, laugh, or speak may consciously or subconsciously try to hide this by covering their mouth with their hand or by intentionally not lifting their upper lip.

In these clinical situations, teeth looking too short or teeth that appear too long, there are dental procedures that can be used to put your gum tissue in its normal, proper location in order to fix the problem.

## GUMS AND COSMETIC DENTISTRY

You know, patients do not usually come to see a dentist and say, "Can you check out my gums?" No, they come to my office and want to know, "Can you make my teeth look nicer?" That is all right – I do not expect the patient to be an expert on gum disease and gum location and to know, without being educated about it, that the right thing to do is secure the foundation of your teeth – the gums – before trying to do any work on their teeth appearance.

Dentists have an ethical obligation to inform you about your complete oral health. A good dentist should be honest enough to inform you: "Look, there is no point in you investing your time and hard-earned money in, say, tooth whitening, if you have gum disease that, untreated, could make you lose those nice, white teeth. So first, let us take care of any gum disease issues, and then we can talk about cosmetic procedures". That is the dentist's job as a medical professional, to take the time to educate you, the patient, so that you can make intelligently informed choices.

And when dentists and their staff do that – make a concerted effort to educate patients so that they understand basic concepts to include gum disease and recession – then the patient not only gets what they really want but also what they need to achieve a great-looking smile.

Dentists should not be talking about merely the appearance of individual teeth, but about the total look of your smile, which includes the appearance of your gums in relation to the lips and face. Fortunately, more and more dentists are taking a holistic approach, discussing how your overall health affects the health of your teeth and gums – not their appearance.

In my professional opinion, all cosmetic dental procedures should begin with an evaluation and appropriate treatment of your gums before treating the teeth. The bottom line is that cosmetic procedures such as veneers or orthodontic treatments should not be undertaken unless your gums and supporting bone are already healthy or after successful gum treatments.

## COSMETIC GUM TREATMENTS - CORRECTING THE "SHORT TEETH" LOOK

In addition to treating gum disease, I also perform cosmetic gum procedures. One of the most common cosmetic treatments for gums is correcting the condition where a patient's gum tissue is covering too much of the bottom portion of his or her teeth, giving the appearance of having short or tiny-looking teeth.

Your teeth come out of the bone of your skull – specifically, your jaw bone. When you are a small child you have "baby" teeth, and then your adult teeth follow those teeth. This occurs in two phases: active and passive. The active eruption phase is the teeth coming out of the bone, the part we are all familiar with, your adult teeth coming in to replace your lost "baby teeth."

But there is also a passive eruption phase that is the gum tissue migrating – moving – into its final, mature location around the neck of each tooth.

When that passive phase occurs correctly, the tooth is properly exposed above your gum line, and everything looks how it is supposed to. However, when the gum tissue does not settle down properly around the neck of the tooth, an excessive amount of gum tissue is covering part of the enamel of your teeth, making them appear short. This tends to make adults, when they smile or speak, look like they have child-sized teeth.

In layman's terms, this condition is often referred to as having a "gummy smile" which can be corrected with a simple procedure called esthetic crown lengthening. That phrase sounds like a mouthful, I know, but it is really a fairly simple procedure, designed to make sure the teeth appear to be properly proportioned in relation to the gums.

The periodontist first examines the teeth and takes all the necessary measurements. The front six to ten teeth, depending on how wide the patient can smile, are anesthetized. The procedure begins with a gingivectomy, in which the periodontist removes a precise number of millimeters of gum tissue on each tooth involved, based on the measurements taken previously. Then, the periodontist re-contours the bone, creating the ideal relationship of bone to gum and tooth. Esthetic crown lengthening is a common procedure performed before veneers and crowns are fabricated and during, or at the conclusion of, orthodontics, i.e., braces.

I recommend that patients find a board-certified periodontist who is always up to date on cutting-edge dental technology. Having a skilled dental professional who utilizes the latest surgical techniques makes all the difference in the world as far as having the absolute best clinical outcome and overall patient experience with minimal discomfort. Newer, less-invasive dental procedures continue to be target of the most innovations in periodontics.

Highly skilled periodontists (and dentists) are also gentle with their approaches. They can do extensive dental work on your teeth and gums without leaving you in a lot of pain when the anesthetic wears off. In the case of esthetic crown lengthening, the patient usually leaves the periodontist's office with a few stitches that will dissolve over the next couple of weeks. Then the patient will come back a few weeks later so that the periodontist can take a look and make sure that the gums have healed properly, and that the patient has gotten the look they want for their smile.

One of the greatest benefits of the esthetic crown lengthening procedure is that it is something a periodontist can do in about an hour and then the patient can see instantaneous results.

The cost for a cosmetic treatment like this, depending mostly on how many teeth are involved, usually runs from two to three thousand dollars. That is a fair price considering orthodontic treatment can cost double to move teeth. There is always the question of whether insurance will cover this procedure. However, every plan, and every insurance company, is different. Typically, dental insurance, like medical insurance, does not cover cosmetic procedures. If a patient has to cover the majority of the costs themselves, most dental offices will offer them a number of payment options to lessen the financial burden.

## COSMETIC GUM TREATMENTS - CORRECTING GUM RECESSION

Unlike excessive gums, gum recession is when the teeth appear longer than they ideally should be, usually as a result of periodontitis, although there can be other causes, such as a patient having thin gum tissue. The quality and quantity of the gum tissue plays a vital role in preventing or exacerbating gum recession. The position of your teeth in relation to your jawbone can cause the "long in the tooth" look, too.

In some cases, this condition can be caused by hard tooth brushing over a period of years, especially with hard or firm bristle toothbrushes. Some patients, who brush their teeth and gums too aggressively, inadvertently cause the gum tissue to move down the tooth and expose the roots. This is one of the reasons it is always recommended for patients to utilize soft bristled toothbrushes since medium and hard bristled toothbrushes can accelerate gum recession. Basically, there are a number of things that, as people naturally age, can cause gum recession and elongated teeth.

One contributing factor for gum recession is being in orthodontics or having a history of orthodontic treatment. Teeth usually erupt where the bone is the thickest. Often, the spot where the bone is the thickest is not the precise spot where the teeth need to be in order to be perfectly aligned.

As the orthodontist attempts to align the teeth and put them into the correct location, he or she begins moving the teeth outward towards the lips and cheeks. For many patients, the bone and gum tissue is significantly thinner towards the lips and cheeks. In any event, it is not uncommon for patients who have had braces to start experiencing gum recession, even though they do not actually have any active gum disease.

I am very much in favor of using a multi-disciplinary approach to cosmetic dentistry, where general dentistry practitioners, along with appropriate specialists, all work together to evaluate patients and design the best possible plan for each individual.

Let me illustrate how that works in practice. For example, sometimes with patients who receive orthodontics treatment, the orthodontist will have a periodontist perform preventive gum grafting procedures if the patient has noticeably thin gum tissue or the tissue has already receded. Gum grafting prior to or during orthodontic treatment can prevent gum recession problems from occurring in the future.

## GUM DISEASE CONDITIONS THAT REQUIRE TREATMENT

There are two basic types of gum disease – gingivitis and periodontitis. Gingivitis shows up as inflamed, irritated, or bleeding gums. The more serious kind of gum disease is periodontitis, where you have actually had some bone loss around your teeth. Periodontitis can be mild, moderate, or severe and lead to tooth loss.

Periodontal disease is very common. The American Academy of Periodontology states that one out of two adults over the age of thirty have some form of periodontitis. Some patients are born with a genetic predisposition to develop periodontal disease. Others may develop it because of poor oral hygiene, having comorbid systemic diseases, and/or because they use tobacco products.

If you have been going to your dentist regularly for several years and receiving adequate treatment all along, then there is a good chance that you have been able to catch early on any gum disease that may have developed, and successfully treat it with non-surgical procedures. In that case, if you start thinking about some cosmetic dental work that you may want to have done, then you are probably in a position to go right ahead with getting cosmetic dental work after discussing treatment options with your dentist and deciding on a treatment option.

On the other hand, with a new patient, especially one who has not been receiving regular dental care for a number of years, there is a good chance that the dentist will need to address some gum disease problems before being in a position to do any cosmetic work the patient wants.

Performing a complete assessment of the condition of a patient's gums, which includes full mouth probe depths and radiographs, allows a periodontist to determine whether they have gingivitis or periodontitis. If the patient has gingivitis, that can usually be corrected with non-surgical treatment, and then he or she can go ahead with orthodontic or other cosmetic treatment after a couple of months.

With periodontitis, if there is only mild bone loss, then the nonsurgical procedure of choice is scaling and root planning, what patients may know as "deep cleaning". It is a little more than your typical cleaning when you go to the dentist. The main difference is that the dentist will give you a local anesthetic for the deep cleaning on those teeth that have mild periodontal disease.

A deep cleaning treatment usually takes about two, two-hour appointments that allow adequate time for dental anesthesia and for the hygienists to do a thorough job. In addition to removing bacteria with the cleaning, the entire dental team will spend a great deal of time educating the patient, so that they can change their dental care habits and hopefully avoid ever getting more severe forms of periodontitis. This is crucial to changing the dental habits of patients and needs to be reinforced at future appointments.

I tell patients all the time that every single tooth could have a completely different periodontal diagnosis. You might have a completely healthy tooth, next to a tooth with gingivitis, next to a tooth with severe periodontitis. And in all of those situations, the treatment is different.

However, if you have moderate to severe periodontitis that typically requires a surgical procedure, you will probably be treated then maintained for a period of six to twelve months depending on the specific surgery and course of treatment. It is important to take care of periodontitis, because otherwise – if you do not get the gums and bone around your teeth healthy – then whatever cosmetic treatment you receive may be a waste of your time and money.

I always try to make sure patients do understand this: It is crucial to first make sure the supporting foundation is in good shape before investing money in cosmetic procedures to give you that really beautiful smile. Again, it may be helpful to recall the analogy of a photo and a frame. Your "photo" (teeth) is never going to look like you want it to if the picture "frame" (gums) is seriously damaged.

## RISKS OF UNTREATED GUM RECESSION

It is important to understand what a potentially serious problem gum recession is if left untreated. If you have gum recession and do not get the proper treatment for it, you are at a significantly increased risk for tooth sensitivity, root cavities, and overall tooth loss.

The greater the amount of recession, the more likely you are to ultimately lose a tooth – or multiple teeth. The exposure of the root surface of a tooth leaves you much more vulnerable to getting root cavities – cavities that occur on the bottom part of the exposed tooth, above the gum line.

Root cavities are particularly dangerous, as compared to a cavity in the body or top portion of a tooth, because the cavity is eating away the structure that holds the tooth in place in your jaw, and that is why tooth loss is a real possibility.

As we age, many adults develop systemic diseases that require medications. Unfortunately, one of the many side effects of these medications is decreasing the amount of saliva creating a condition called dry mouth. Dry mouth, while annoying to the patient, can be detrimental to the teeth – especially if the teeth have experienced gingival recession increasing the chance of root cavities.

Root cavities are different than regular cavities. Most people are probably familiar with the term "enamel", which is the protective coating that usually covers each of your teeth. Enamel is pretty resistant to cavities, although of course, patients with poor oral hygiene and poor diet can get cavities through your tooth enamel.

The main reason root cavities differ from cavities in the in the enamel is the gum recession has exposed a different part of the tooth – the cementum-covered root, a part of the tooth that is not normally exposed. What is different about the root is that there is no protective enamel covering on the root part of your teeth. The enamel is designed to protect the upper, outer portion of your teeth, and the gum tissue is supposed to protect the root of the tooth. But if your gums recede, then that protection for the root of your tooth is not there. Once you start to acquire a root cavity, the cavity gets worse much quicker, the damage advances more rapidly. After a very short period of time, the damage can quickly reach the point where there is nothing your dentist can do to save the tooth, and it has to be removed.

I cannot stress enough that if you have gum recession, you need to get it treated as soon as possible. Once you lose an adult tooth, it is not coming back. This is why it is critical for you to visit a dentist every six months. The main early warning sign of gum disease is bleeding of the gums. But one thing I should mention is that people who use tobacco products may not show that early warning sign. That is because tobacco products constrict your blood vessels, which makes you less prone to bleeding. That is another reason I tell my patients that everyone should be evaluated at a dental office twice a year.

## TREATMENT FOR GUM RECESSION WITH PERIODONTAL PLASTIC SURGERY

The traditional way to treat gum recession is by using time-tested gingival grafting technique that has been around for many years. This treatment involves harvesting a free-gingival graft or the underlying connective tissue from the patient's palate, to use as donor tissue, which is then sutured or stitched into place in the area of the gum where there is gum recession. The patient's natural gum tissue that is below the recession is stitched up over the top of the grafted area.

The advantage of this technique is that the dentist is using the patient's own tissue for the procedure, transplanting the patient's gum tissue from one location to another.

But the disadvantage is that there is usually multiple teeth requiring treatment, and there is only so much tissue available from the palate that can be transplanted. So it is difficult, if not impossible, to get enough tissue to completely take care of everything. Furthermore, harvesting tissue from the palate causes discomfort for the patient, which is something periodontists really try to avoid nowadays.

If you have several teeth requiring treatment for gum recession, then this traditional gum grafting approach is neither realistic nor practical. There is a limited amount of tissue to work with, plus, it would take multiple visits and procedures over several months or years, something most patients are unwilling to do.

Because of the limitations with using the traditional gum grafting procedure, the mid-1990s brought about a new approach in the treatment of gum recession. No longer was there an absolute requirement for harvesting the patient's own tissue. In 1997, LifeCell™ introduced acellular dermal matrix (i.e., Alloderm®, etc.) for dental applications.

Researchers were able to acquire larger amounts of donor skin tissue in the same way that other organs, such as bone, is acquired. Skin is harvested from people who have designated themselves as donors upon becoming deceased. Once a certified tissue bank has verified through testing that the donor tissue free of diseases (e.g., viruses, etc.), the outer epithelium is removed and the underlying dermis and basement membrane are prepared in such a way that cells are removed but the blood vessels, collagen, elastin, etc., remain. This allows the graft to act as a scaffold for the normal tissue remolding after surgical placement.

And so now, instead of taking tissue from the patient's palate, a periodontist can open up a package of sterilized acellular dermal matrix tissue. The donor tissue graft is prepared then stitched into place and then the patient's gums are stitched up over the top of the graft. This innovation allows periodontists to treat large areas of recession in a single visit with much less discomfort for the patient.

Recently, a newer, less invasive treatment approach for treating gum recession was developed, and this new procedure is now one of our preferred treatment methods. It is called the Chao Pinhole® Surgical Technique (PST™), named for the developer of this proprietary gum recession treatment – Dr. John Chao, DDS, JD.

The PST™ is great because it is a scalpel-free, suture-free procedure, which makes it very appealing for patients. The creative innovation is that, instead of having to loosen the gum tissue right in between the teeth, the periodontist creates tiny pinholes, four to six per jaw, in the mucous membrane. Then, while utilizing specially designed dental instruments, the periodontist gently tunnels and loosens the gum tissue around the tooth and then slides it up along the neck of the tooth. The last step is to place small non-crossed linked collagen under the papillae and along the neck of the teeth.

While this sounds complex, the important thing to know is that the procedure allows your periodontist to treat recession without doing any cutting or stitching, and so there is only minimal, short-term discomfort or swelling for the patient.

My staff and I were trained at the Chao Pinhole Academy near Pasadena, California in 2016, and we really like how our patients have responded to the treatment. Our patients that have opted for the PST™ experience much less discomfort while at the same time we are able to do an even higher quality job of treating the recession. Empirically, I would estimate that patients heal almost twice as fast, as compared to using the traditional gum grafting technique because the papillae remain intact.

## NEW PERIODONTAL TREATMENTS

There are a variety of periodontal treatments available for you, some surgical and some non-surgical, as well as new ways of treating gum disease. Most of the new treatments that have been developed in the past five to ten years are more effective and less invasive, which means that patients heal faster and do not have to deal with as much discomfort, like the PST™ I mentioned earlier.

If you have some mild to moderate level of gum disease that can be easily taken care of with non-surgical treatment, then that is great because you are probably going to heal pretty quickly and be ready sooner for any cosmetic dental procedure. However, it is still going to be probably at least two or three months before all your tissues are completely healed to the point where you are ready to move forward in getting some cosmetic work done. If you have severe periodontal disease, then that healing period is likely going to take a bit longer, even if the periodontist employs one of the newer, less invasive treatments.

One of the newest and most exciting technologies we have been utilizing in our office for more than five years for treating moderate to severe periodontal disease with a unique dental laser. The device is called a PerioLase®. You can probably tell by the name that it is a type of laser that has been specifically developed to treat moderate to severe periodontal disease.

The PerioLase® was created by Millennium Dental Technologies of Cerritos, California, and, honestly, it is revolutionizing how gum disease is treated worldwide. The PerioLase® is used to perform a specific type of Laser Periodontal Therapy™ called Laser Assisted New Attachment Procedure® or LANAP® for short. With LANAP® it is possible to achieve Laser-Assisted Regeneration™ or LAR™. LANAP® is the only FDA-cleared laser to promote True Regeneration™ of the attachment apparatus (new cementum, new periodontal ligament, and new alveolar bone) on a previously diseased root surface when used specifically in the LANAP® Protocol. My staff and I have been specially certified to utilize the PerioLase® and have found it achieves wonderful results for our patients without the need for a scalpel, bone grafting, or stiches.

## IS GUM DISEASE REVERSIBLE?

A common question patients have is the question, "Is gum disease reversible?"

Gingivitis, the less severe kind of gum disease is completely reversible with a combination of professional dental cleaning and educating the patient on proper dental care, including daily brushing of the gums, flossing, and using oral rinses.

The more severe kind of gum disease, periodontitis, is not generally reversible without surgical intervention but it can be effectively treated – depending on the severity.

With the most severe cases, there may be nothing your dentist can do to save the tooth, and in those instances, the proper treatment involves talking about tooth removal and tooth replacement such as a dental implant.

## LIFE-CHANGING TREATMENT

Let me tell you about one patient I treated, whose case illustrates what a transformational difference getting treated for gum disease can make in a person's life.

This was actually a cosmetic case. Maria was in her late twenties when she was referred to me. She had significant gum recession after undergoing orthodontic treatment. Her chief complaint is that, because of her "long tooth" condition, she no longer smiled. She said she was always self-conscious about the way she spoke and laughed because she could see how long her teeth were.

As you can gather, in Maria's situation, the condition of her teeth in relation to her gums was having a severely negative effect on how she lived her daily life and interacted with people. It affected her personal relationships; it affected how she acted at work, and indeed her entire life. Because Maria was so self-conscious and embarrassed about her smile, she was reluctant to socialize with people at all. This was all attributable to gum recession.

We performed extensive gum grafting for her, and the difference was nothing short of miraculous. When she came back to my office for a checkup one month later, she was actually in tears because she was so happy about having regained her self-confidence. It was really remarkable – her whole life changed dramatically for the better in less than a month.

Maria is not alone. I have treated many patients with the same or similar oral conditions. People may not realize what a difference a beautiful smile can make, but I would argue that by getting the proper treatment, you can make your smile, and in effect, your whole face, look 10 or 20 years younger. Periodontal plastic surgery can boost your self-confidence and self-esteem, and that shows through. These procedures have the potential to change everything about a person – how they carry themselves, their facial expressions, and self-confidence.

It can be both shocking and devastating for someone to hear that they have severe periodontal disease. Sometimes certain teeth can be saved, but in some cases, it is recommended to have teeth removed and consider tooth replacement options such as dental implants. Patients need to talk to their dental professional about their options.

As sobering as it may be to hear you need some or all of your teeth removed, we explain the systemic benefits to the patient's overall health. In addition, we discuss tooth replacement options, such as dental implants. We say, "Our goal is to restore balance in your mouth. In time, you will be chewing food like you used to and have a beautiful smile." Restoring balance to chewing while delivering optimal dental esthetics is the ultimate goal for everyone.

I always take the time to explain to patients that it is really important to get treatment because severe periodontal disease can put their whole systemic health at risk. The associations between periodontal disease and systemic diseases – known as the oral-systemic link – are well documented. Your overall systemic health and your oral health often times run hand-in-hand.

One of the most common connections is with diabetes including those pre-diabetic (i.e., glucose intolerance, etc.). People with uncontrolled or poorly controlled diabetes tend to have much more frequent gum disease issues and severity. Of equal importance is that untreated periodontal disease can exacerbate their diabetes condition. Both must be treated to improve the quality and longevity of life for these patients.

Pregnant women with periodontal disease have a higher chance of having a preterm low birth weight baby. Studies show that women that get their periodontal disease under control earlier during their pregnancy have a better chance of their baby being born full term. Also, men with periodontal disease have much higher rates of erectile dysfunction (ED). Studies show that once these men have their periodontal disease effectively treated, most will experience fewer ED issues.

People with active periodontal disease are much more likely to have problems throughout their bodies. Inflammatory mediators and bacteria are constantly entering their bloodstream while targeting the heart and brain. Those with untreated periodontal disease have an increased risk for both heart attack and stroke, as they are all comorbid risk factors in the overall health of a patient. Educating people on the oral-systemic link is a must for each dentist and periodontist. Only well-informed people can be expected to make educated, sometimes life-altering decisions that may affect more than his or her teeth but may also prolong the quality and quantity of life.

Today, most of our patients are very thankful when we can use less invasive procedures, such as the PerioLase® or the Chao Pinhole® Surgical Technique before things become too severe. My patients are thankful and happy not only that we saved their teeth but also because we were able to take a more conservative approach than were possible just a few years ago.

Again, I want to stress that the most important thing is to see your dentist regularly, so that he or she has the opportunity to recognize, at an early stage, any developing problem with gum disease. If you only have gingivitis, then your dentist and dental hygienist can completely treat the areas and give you the knowledge and skills needed to take the best possible care of your teeth to prevent any future problems.

If you have taken the time to read this book, my message to you is simple. I want you to have the best-looking, most attractive smile possible, for your entire life. And there is no reason you cannot have that. In my ideal world, everyone gets proper education on taking care of their teeth and gums, in addition to visiting their dentist twice a year. If your dentist diagnoses you with any form of periodontal disease, it is recommended to see a periodontist as soon as possible. Together, the dentist and periodontist can come up with a plan to restore your dental health and, in many cases, improve your quality of life.

# About Bryan P. Kalish, DDS, MS

Implant & Laser Periodontal Surgery Center
SouthwestImplantSurgery.com

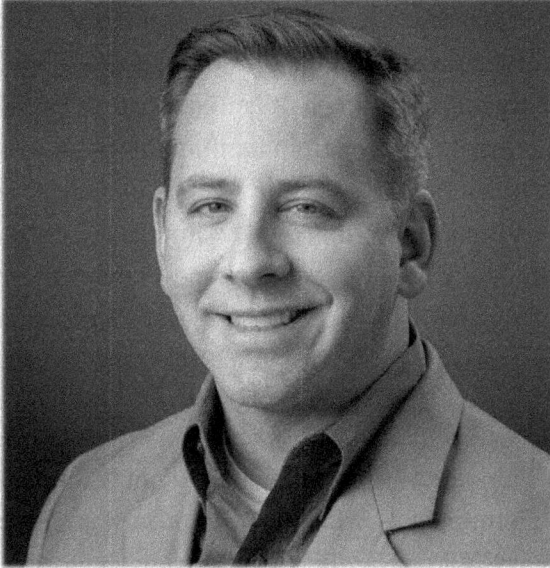

Dr. Bryan P. Kalish has been providing exceptional patient care for nearly a decade and, since his recent retirement from the military, has become part of the El Paso dental community.

As a former periodontal and implant surgery instructor in the United States Army, Dr. Kalish attained the rank of full-bird colonel and received numerous awards and commendations including: the US Army Dental Corps Chief's Exceptional Service and Leadership Award, the US Army Surgeon General's "A" Proficiency Designator, which is recognized as the highest level of professional achievement in the US Army Medical Department, and the Legion of Merit for exceptionally meritorious service.

Dr. Kalish specializes in dental implants, bone grafting, and the use of laser and cosmetic periodontal practices. He also specializes in cosmetic lip and cheek injectable fillers, therapeutic Botox to treat TMD and myofascial pain, and the creation of oral sleep appliances.

Dr. Kalish amasses over 100 hours per year of ongoing training. He also travels frequently to demonstrate the most cutting-edge surgical techniques at seminars all over the world, working with other dentists to train them in the latest technology available to help patients receive the highest quality dental care. He has received certificates in Kybella Chin Treatments, Pinhole Surgical Technique, Lip Augmentation and Platelet Rich Plasma Injections, Advanced Botox and Dermal Fillers, and Laser-Assisted New Attachment Procedure® (LANAP) Evolution 5 Proficiency.

Dr. Kalish graduated from college and dental school through the Six-Year Combined BA/DDS program at the University of Missouri – Kansas City (UMKC). He practiced general dentistry in the Army for four years before specializing in dental implants and periodontal surgery. He has worked with patients in Thailand, Korea, Mongolia, Germany, Italy, and Iraq. Today, his passion is to work with patients in the southwestern United States, many of whom travel great distances to receive care from him.

A few of his professional accolades include Fellow, Institute for Advanced Laser Dentistry; Fellow, International College of Dentists; Member of the Order of Military Medical Merit; Master in the College of Sedation in Dentistry; Past-President of the European Association of Military Periodontists; Board-Certified Diplomate of the American Board of Periodontology; and membership in the American Board of Periodontology, American Academy of Periodontology, American Academy of Dental Sleep Medicine, American Dental Association, Texas Dental Association, El Paso District Dental Society, Institute for

Advanced Laser Dentistry, and International Academy of Facial Aesthetics. He is licensed to practice dentistry is Texas and New Mexico.

# IMMEDIATE MAKEOVER WITH DENTAL VENEERS

One popular cosmetic dental treatment that I specialize in is the application of dental veneers – also known as porcelain veneers or porcelain laminates. Veneers are very thin, custom-fitted shells that are bonded to the front of your teeth in order to improve your smile by changing the color, shape, or the size of your teeth.

The application of veneers can bring about a remarkable transformation in the appearance of your teeth. Let me tell you about one patient I helped. This was one of my first cases where I used veneers, almost 20 years ago. My patient's name was Michael. Michael first came to see me when he was just 17 years old, right after having his braces removed after wearing them for **five years**. The braces straightened his teeth, but Michael still wasn't happy with the appearance of his smile, because of a problem known as pegged laterals or peg teeth.

Peg teeth are very skinny and lack good, square or rounded corners. In short, they resemble pegs and there are noticeable spaces between the teeth.

Michael was very self-conscious about the appearance of his teeth and became one of those people who automatically covers their mouth with their hand when they smile so people won't see their teeth. It was very sad. Here he'd endured having braces since he was 12 years old, for **five years**, but when he finally removed his braces, he was still embarrassed by the appearance of his teeth.

The orthodontist who did Michael's braces referred him me to discuss what cosmetic procedure we could perform to get rid of those spaces and give Michael the attractive smile he wanted.

After looking at Michael's teeth, I recommended teeth whitening as a good first step to brighten his smile after having the braces on for so long. I knew porcelain veneers would be a perfect way to fix his peg teeth; and they were.

The happy ending to this story is that after we put the porcelain veneers over his upper teeth, getting rid of the spaces between teeth and giving his teeth a fuller, more squared off look, Michael was voted as having the "best smile" in his high school that year. That really made him smile. There was no more covering his mouth with a hand – Michael was proud to show people his teeth. The bonus was how much self-confidence Michael built up due to his super-attractive smile. He sent me a picture of his high school yearbook photo, and told me about being voted "best smile". I was so happy that I helped him look better and feel better about himself. Having a great smile and the self-confidence that goes with it can make a significant difference in personal and professional experiences.

There's a second happy ending to Michael's story. I got a phone call from him about four years ago, right before an important job interview he had. He told me he'd been playing basketball and caught an elbow in the mouth that popped one of his veneers off. It was already evening, and his job interview was scheduled for the next morning. He arrived at my office around midnight, and I quickly cemented the veneer back on. He got the job! That's the kind of difference that looking in the mirror and knowing you have a great smile can make in your life; it boosts your self-esteem.

## WHAT ARE VENEERS AND WHAT ARE THEY USED FOR

Dental veneers are a very simple cosmetic dental product. They are usually made of porcelain or resin, and they are essentially a shell that we custom make and bond to the front of the tooth. Veneers are used to give your teeth a best possible shape, size, length, width, or color – and therefore can be used as a whitening treatment.

In fact, you can use veneers to change the appearance of your teeth in virtually any way you want. Getting veneers can fix a cosmetic problem like gaps between teeth or tooth discoloration. The end goal, whatever the specific reason for getting veneers, is for you to have a better, more attractive smile.

Getting veneers can also help you look younger and healthier, because brighter, whiter, more perfectly formed teeth are associated with youth and good health. The process of aging wears down your teeth, causes loss of part of the hard enamel protective coating, increases staining of the teeth, and changes tooth alignment. Veneers can do wonders and help you look younger by lengthening or widening your teeth, which provides important support for your lips and cheeks that can diminish as you get older.

Veneers are commonly used to fix chipped or broken teeth, though in some cases, veneers are used to restore the appearance of perfectly straight teeth without having to get braces. Some people have a habit of grinding their teeth in their sleep, which wears down the teeth over time.

Veneers offer an easy solution for creating an ideal smile. Veneers are custom made for the purpose of giving the patient the smile they want. For example, some people prefer the corners of their teeth more rounded, while others prefer them more squared off. We can create veneers to give you whatever look you prefer.

## TYPES OF VENEERS

In addition to the traditional porcelain or composite resin veneers, there are more types of veneers to choose from today. Porcelain veneers are aesthetically superior and do a better job of reflecting light, because porcelain is similar to natural tooth enamel, and is a better choice for maintaining whiter teeth because porcelain is better at resisting staining.

Composite resin, while a bit less expensive, isn't as bright-white to begin with and tends to absorb stains over time. The resin is used a lot less frequently these days.

Technological advances in cosmetic dentistry mean that there are new materials to choose from, such as lithium disilicate or zirconia. These more modern veneers are known as CAD/CAM, which refers to the fact that they are crafted with computer-assisted design (CAD) and computer-assisted milling (CAM) materials.

The CAM materials have the advantage of being up to 10 times stronger than porcelain veneers, which means they are more durable and last longer. Compared to porcelain veneers, these new materials are a lot closer to having the strength and durability of natural teeth.

The newer computer-assisted crowns made with materials like zirconia are replacing traditional porcelain veneers as the favored veneer material. One advantage zirconia offers is durability in cases where patients grind or clench their teeth a lot. Porcelain is prone to fracture, whereas these newer materials can stand up to grinding or clenching without breaking or wearing down.

However, porcelain veneers are still, in most cases, the most aesthetically pleasing. They're closest to being perfect, natural, bright, and white in appearance.

The best veneer choice for you will depend on the specific cosmetic treatment that you're looking for, how many teeth are going to be covered with veneers, and the kind of smile you want. Just be aware that there are many options available, so be sure to discuss all the possible choices with your dentist when you talk about getting veneers.

## PREPLESS VENEERS

A special, very limited use of veneers is a treatment known as prepless veneers. Prepless veneers are exactly what the name implies – veneers that are bonded to your teeth without doing any work on the existing tooth structure.

Prepless veneers are typically used for very minor cosmetic changes like improving the color of teeth that may have become stained or discolored over time. Prepless veneers do offer the advantage of being relatively inexpensive compared to more complex cosmetic treatments with veneers, since all they require is taking an impression of your teeth, then bonding the veneers.

Because prepless veneers are generally less aesthetically pleasing and more prone to popping off, breaking and needing to be replaced, I don't usually recommend that option; though in some cases it can be an appropriate treatment.

If you're thinking about having prepless veneers, I would recommend going to a dentist with known experience and skill. Prepless veneers are very thin and challenging to get the coloration right. The dentist must blend in shades of color from the cement used in the bonding, and it takes a great deal of skill to become an expert in that technique.

Prepless veneers are probably the most difficult type of veneer to deliver, so you need a dentist who has the necessary training and skill to perform that delicate work.

## NORMAL PROCEDURE FOR GETTING VENEERS

Although veneers are a much less complex cosmetic dental treatment than procedures such as dental implants, they usually require a couple of visits to your dentist.

The first visit is the consultation or examination, where your dentist examines your teeth, usually takes X-rays, perhaps takes an impression of your teeth, and then discusses the various treatment options, so you can map out a plan for your treatment together. When you're consulting with your dentist, make sure to communicate as clearly as you can, exactly what kind of cosmetic effect you're looking for. For example, if having very white teeth or teeth shaped a certain way (squared or rounded) are very important to you, make sure your dentist is aware of that. Knowing precisely what you want will help your dentist in selecting the most appropriate materials and "smile design" to give you the exact kind of smile you desire.

The actual treatment typically requires two visits. During the first visit, your dentist will prepare the teeth that are to be veneered, and take an impression or mold of your teeth. A small portion of the tooth structure must be removed to get the proper aesthetic look when the veneer is applied. A very small amount of the tooth enamel is removed – usually about 1/2 millimeter, which matches the thickness of the tooth with the thickness of the veneer. That way you don't end up with teeth that are unnaturally thick or that don't match the thickness of your other teeth that are not receiving veneers. The goal is to make sure that all your teeth remain properly proportional to each other in size.

Your dentist then sends your impressions to a dental laboratory that custom crafts your veneers to precisely fit your existing teeth. It usually takes a couple of weeks for your dentist to get the newly made veneers from the laboratory, at which point you come in for your final visit to get the veneers applied (bonded) to your teeth.

Before the actual bonding, your dentist will fit the veneers in place on your teeth to check the fit and appearance. The veneers may need some minor adjustments (trimming) to create the perfect fit for each tooth. The color of the veneer can also be adjusted using a different shade of cement for the bonding. In the final preparation of bonding your veneers, your teeth will be cleaned and then etched, a process that slightly roughens the surface of the tooth in order to get the strongest bond.

Finally, the veneer is bonded to your tooth using a primer, a special cement bonding agent, and an ultraviolet light that activates certain chemicals in the bonding cement, creating a permanent resin that should hold the veneer solidly in place for decades.

After your veneers are applied, the dentist will again check the look of your teeth and your bite and can make some final adjustments if necessary to get everything just right.

It's a good idea to ask your dentist about a follow-up visit a couple of weeks after delivery, to check the veneers and to make sure the veneers aren't irritating your gums. When veneers are first applied, just like crowns, there will be some minor irritation of your gums, but if your veneers are formed and fitted properly, the irritation should subside within a few days.

## CAN VENEERS DAMAGE YOUR TEETH?

Some patients are concerned about removing a thin slice of tooth enamel to make room for the veneer to be applied. The fact is, that some enamel is worn away just in the ordinary course of eating and drinking, especially if you regularly drink very acidic beverages such as coffee or tea. The normal wear and tear of chewing or grinding gradually removes some of the structure of a tooth.

On average, your teeth have about three millimeters of protective enamel covering over the live part of the tooth, the dentin and the nerve. So, if as your dentist I remove 1/2 millimeter, or even a millimeter and a half, there's still a layer of protection for the nerve and dentin. Plus, the veneer itself offers a layer of protection. Getting veneers doesn't effectively make your teeth any weaker or more prone to cavities.

There can be some instances where a patient has already lost a lot of enamel, such as from gradual acid erosion, injury, or grinding, and therefore the shaving of enamel to make room for a veneer is occurring much closer to the nerve.

There are rare occasions where there can be nerve inflammation that makes it necessary to do a root canal. It is likely that part of the reason you're seeking cosmetic dental treatment is because you've lost some enamel, chipped, or worn down your teeth. There is a small risk that a root canal may be necessary to avoid oversensitivity or nerve inflammation, because there may not be enough solid tooth structure to apply a veneer.

If your tooth enamel is already worn down significantly when you get veneers, you may find that you have more sensitivity to hot or cold beverages.

The important thing is to make sure that your dentist fully explains the procedure to you, and that you have the knowledge you need to make an informed decision to accept the risks.

In my 20 years, I've probably done around 30,000 crowns and veneers, and out of all those tens of thousands, only a handful of times have we had to do a root canal afterward. Understand that when that happens, it's primarily a result of wear and tear, or damage that's already occurred to the tooth, not a result of applying veneers.

Again, that only happens in a very small percentage of cases, but it is something that I discuss with patients beforehand to make sure they understand everything before I give them that life-changing smile.

## STRENGTH AND DURABILITY OF VENEERS

One of the real positives of veneers is that they are durable and can last up to 25 years or more, if the patient takes good care of them. The most common reason for a veneer to come off is an injury.

I had a patient once with beautiful veneers on her front teeth. She got up in the middle of the night to get a glass of water, and because she couldn't see the glass in the dark as she brought it up to her mouth, she hit her front teeth with the edge of the glass and cracked her two front veneers and had to have them replaced.

That's the kind of thing that usually causes a veneer to crack or pop off. Outside of trauma like that, veneers can easily last for decades.

If you compare the strength of veneers to natural teeth, porcelain veneers are somewhat more brittle, but the new materials we're using to make veneers, like zirconium, are almost as structurally sound as a natural tooth. Therefore, they can last longer and handle a lot more pressure or trauma. They also fare better than porcelain veneers against grinding and clenching. I usually recommend choosing the newer, stronger materials for patients who grind and clench.

If a patient grinds or clenches a lot in their sleep, that intense muscle activity has the capability of fracturing porcelain veneers. Therefore, if you grind or clench your teeth, you can help protect your veneers by getting a night guard or other tooth guard appliance to wear when you sleep. Protecting your veneers with the appropriate appliance will help them look and feel great, and last longer.

## COST OF VENEERS

The cost of veneers can vary considerably depending on what part of the country you live in, but the cost typically ranges somewhere between $1,500 and $3,000 per tooth, or per veneer. In most areas, other than places where the cost of living is high, like New York or San Francisco, the average cost is about $1,500 to $2,000 per tooth. There usually isn't a significant cost difference between porcelain veneers and the newer materials, so it is ideal to choose the most appropriate material for your individual case.

Unfortunately, getting veneers usually isn't covered by most insurance plans.

Workmen's compensation or insurance will usually only pay for veneers when veneers are the best option to restore teeth broken in an accident. But like other cosmetic treatments that may not be covered by insurance, most good dentists will work with you to help you arrange financing or set up a payment plan with payment installments rather than paying the full cost all at once.

## How Many Veneers Does it Take to Make a Great Smile?

A common question I get from patients is how many veneers does it usually take to create that life-changing smile. The answer to that question is open-ended, because it depends on the individual patient. Some patients come in with a general desire to improve the look of their teeth and their smile, and so we'll explore all the various options in terms of treatments, types of material, and risks versus benefits. Some patients arrive with a photo from a magazine of an actor, actress or model who has a great smile and say, "I want my smile to look like that."

With a clear picture of your desired smile, your dentist can give you a smile evaluation illustrating the differences between your current smile and the smile you want, and present you with treatment options and a smile plan design.

As far as how many veneers you need to get your desired smile, it depends on what you're trying to do. Do we need to widen your smile? Lengthen teeth? Cover up receding gums? One of the factors that determine how many veneers are needed is the width of your smile. Some people have a narrow smile where you only see a few teeth, while other people have a very wide smile where you can see all their teeth, including their first molars.

For example, the actress Halle Berry, who happens to be one of the most frequently requested smile designs, has a very wide smile. So, depending on smile width, a patient might need eight veneers, or they might need only four. Some patients may just need two, if they already have a nice, bright smile, with wide teeth. A lot of patients get veneers on just their two front upper teeth, because those are the teeth that most commonly get chipped in an accident.

Patients with narrower teeth or with gaps between their teeth typically end up getting either four or eight veneers done. Four is the most common. When you consult with your dentist, they can make wax models to show you what the new teeth will look like.

Some dentists use Photoshop to show how having four or eight veneers will change your smile. Seeing possible results before applying veneers makes it easier for you and your dentist to determine how many veneers you may want or need.

Veneers are most commonly done on the upper teeth, but there are instances where putting veneers on the lower teeth can produce an amazing transformation in someone's smile. In cases of grinding and clenching, where the bottom teeth have been worn down, veneers or crowns may be needed to provide lip support.

Getting both upper and lower veneers can restore what we call your vertical bite, creating an astounding transformation and making you appear younger and healthier. When your lip support is restored, your lips will look fuller and more youthful. Your facial wrinkles will be markedly diminished, and the height or length of your teeth will be restored to what it was when you were 18 to 20 years old.

There are a lot of people who think they need a cosmetic procedure like Botox injections, when a well-done set of veneers will get rid of those wrinkles and make them look 20 years younger. A good cosmetic dentist can help support the inside structure of your mouth and make those creases and wrinkles vanish.

I've helped truck drivers who, because they're often stressed out while doing their job, tend to grind their teeth while they're driving. I can build their bite structure back up, and then recommend a daytime mouth guard when they're driving to prevent them from grinding their teeth down again.

Another possible benefit of getting veneers is getting rid of headaches and facial pain. There are a lot of people who have chronic headaches or facial pain, and don't realize that the cause of it is the fact that their bite has been altered by grinding or clenching. As a result, facial nerves are being pinched and causing pain.

## COMPARING VENEERS TO TEETH WHITENING TREATMENTS

When trying to resolve stained or discolored teeth, one alternative treatment to veneers is teeth whitening. The primary difference between these two treatments for teeth whitening purposes is that veneers provide a more significant and permanent solution.

Teeth whitening treatments, whether using home kits or having them done in a dental office, must be repeated periodically as your teeth begin absorbing stains again.

In contrast, veneers offer a more permanent and durable color change that doesn't have to be repeated, again and again. Your veneers don't absorb stains, and porcelain veneers aren't going to change color or fade.

## ISSUES TO CONSIDER WHEN YOU'RE THINKING ABOUT GETTING VENEERS

Veneers and cosmetic dentistry are an art form that requires technical skills and creativity. If you're thinking about getting veneers, find a dentist who not only has the training and experience but who also appreciates the art of the smile. Any dentist can make a crown or a filling, but when you really want to substantially improve your appearance by getting a dream smile, you need a dentist who can look at details and help you envision what is possible with a few well-done veneers. As mentioned earlier, a lot of people don't know that veneers can give them a great smile and improve the overall appearance of their face.

The first thing you should do is take an honest look at your smile and your face in the mirror and ask yourself if you're truly happy with what you see, or would you feel better about yourself with perfect looking teeth and a terrific smile that makes you look younger, brighter, more attractive, and happier. With the advances in cosmetic dentistry, virtually anyone can have a beautiful, movie-star quality smile.

A good smile design can be a life-changing transformation. It was for Joseph, a patient of mine who was a police officer who had three teeth broken in a struggle in the line of duty. He had never been satisfied with his smile before the incident and he was self-conscious about white blotches or spots on his teeth; most likely caused by fluoride in the water.

When he came to see me, he'd already gone to three other dental offices trying to find a cosmetic dentist to help him fix his broken teeth and get rid of the spots. He tried whitening, but it did not take care of the spots. Joseph was very excited when I spoke with him about veneers for his front upper teeth.

I ended up making those veneers for him back in 2002, and since then we've become close friends. We get together at least once a month. What I notice every time I see him is how young he looks and what a terrific, natural looking smile he has. Since we hang out together, I've had the occasion to hear a lot of people compliment Joseph on his great smile, which is rewarding because Joseph hardly ever smiled before he got his veneers done.

If you knew him before and after his veneers, you'd see a world of difference in his self-confidence and the way he carries himself; and since he's always smiling broadly now, people think of him as one of the friendliest people they know.

Seeing that kind of life-changing transformation in people, beyond merely improving their looks, gives me a great feeling of satisfaction as a provider of cosmetic dentistry.

# ABOUT STEVE TATEVOSSIAN, DDS
King House Dental Group
KingHouseDentalGroup.com

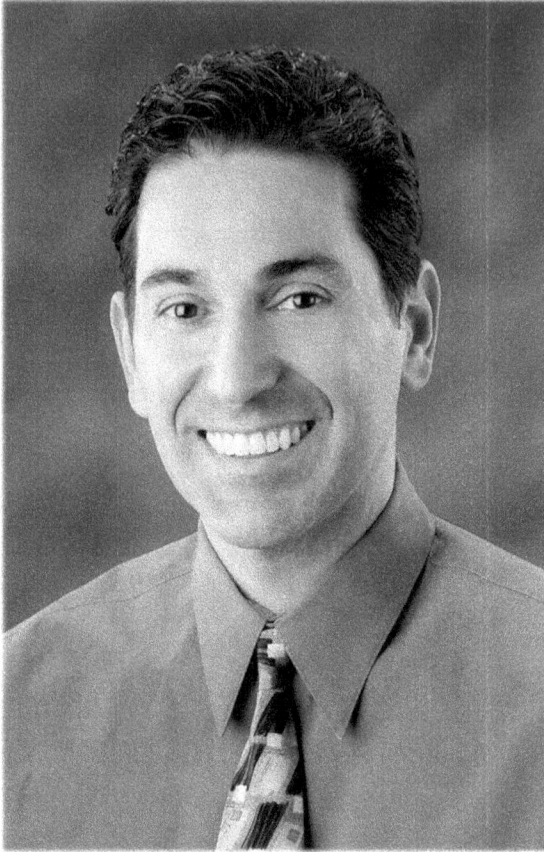

For more than 20 years, Dr. Steve Tatevossian has been ensuring comfortable and professional dental results for his patients.

As a board-certified dentist specializing in general and restorative dentistry for all ages, Dr. Tatevossian and his staff at King House Dental Group combine the highest quality dental care with a compassionate and professional experience. "Dr. T." has spent many years studying the specific challenges associated with dental issues and advocates early detection and pro-active treatment to prevent the need for costly dental procedures. He uses the most advanced technology, including intraoral cameras and digital imaging equipment, to detect and treat dental issues before they become serious problems.

Dr. Tatevossian offers the latest services in cosmetic dentistry, orthodontics, restorations, TMJ disorder treatment, and **sedation dentistry**. Patients who are uncomfortable with having dental work performed can relax in perfect comfort while enjoying the benefits of several forms of sedation. His sedation dentistry practices often allow patients who have been avoiding dental work to take steps to correct issues and problems and have all their dental treatments completed in as little as one visit.

Dr. T. attended the University of California at Riverside (Bachelors in Biology) and graduated from Loma Linda University School of Dentistry in 1996. He was awarded a distinguished Fellowship from the American Academy of Cranio Facial Pain. He is certified and trained in Advanced TMJ and Sleep Therapy, Diagnosis and Treatment of Occlusal Disorders, Treatment of Obstructive Sleep Apnea, and Head and Neck Injections for Craniofacial Pain. Dr. T. is a proud member of the California Dental Association, the Tri- County Dental Association, the American Academy of a Cosmetic Dentistry, the American Academy of Craniofacial Pain, the American Academy of Dental Sleep Medicine and the American Dental Association as well as other professional and community organizations. He has earned numerous awards and hosted his own radio show, *The Dental Detective*, on **AM 1050**. Dr. T. was also the recipient of the *Fox Network Top Doc 2011* award and was nominated for *Best of LA* **KCAL 9** in the General Dentist category.

Throughout his career, Dr. Tatevossian has received numerous distinctions and awards. He has been named as a member of the Advisory Board of the Concorde Career College's Dental Hygiene School. He has also served on the Expert Panel for Lead Physicians; as a member of the Advisory Board for the American Career College's Dental Assisting School and clinical instructor for the college; as a member of the Advisory Board of Western University School of Dentistry; as a Clinical Instructor of Hands on Medical Massage School of Loma Linda; as a clinical instructor at Ashdown College in Redlands specializing in head and neck anatomy and cranial therapy.

Dr. T. and his staff serve patients from the Redlands California area, including Yucaipa, Mentone, Highland, Loma Linda, Colton, Calimesa, San Bernardino and Los Angeles.

# BITING RIGHT IS
# BITING TIGHT

In addition to dental treatments focused on individual teeth, we often have to address structural problems with the smile itself. A crooked smile, or debilitating jaw pain, is often the result of problems with the temporal mandibular joint – commonly referred to by its initials, TMJ. The TMJ is the hinge joint that connects the lower jaw to the skull. Everyone has a right and left TMJ, one on either side of the skull. The TMJ moves every time someone eats or talks, making it one of the most important and frequently used joints in the human body.

Problems with jaw alignment and bite are not strictly an aesthetic problem, but can certainly cause aesthetic and cosmetic concerns for patients. Generally, jaw and bite problems cause pain, and patients in pain often simply don't feel like smiling. The jaw or bite problems affect the quality of their lives and how they feel about themselves, as well as their overall health. Patients who have jaw or bite issues - even patients with straight, white teeth - often avoid smiling.

There's also the possible resulting decay, chipping, breaking, and staining of teeth that can be caused by TMJ issues and drastically affect the way a person's smile looks. Bite and jaw issues can easily affect someone's overall attitude. I've seen many cases where these issues, until they were properly treated, caused mental and emotional problems as well, and just an overall poor quality of life.

Let me try to illustrate what I'm talking about for you with a story about a life-changing treatment for an actual patient of mine.

*This patient's story provides a great example of how treating TMJ issues is not just a matter of correcting functionality, but also about making a real difference in how a patient looks and feels about themselves. The patient was a gentleman who was in his early sixties when he first came to see me. One of the very first things he told me about his overall problem was that he didn't smile much.*

*After the initial examination, I could see that he had a number of chipped and damaged teeth, which was a large contributing factor to his unwillingness to smile. However, he also had substantial jaw and alignment issues. He had limited functionality of both TMJs and experienced clicking, popping, and severe headaches.*

*Part of this patient's treatment involved getting him into a splint that helped to get his jaw muscles in a more comfortable and better-functioning position. It was then that I mentioned additional cosmetic procedures that could be done to correct some of the discoloration and chipping on his upper teeth, as the splint would be covering his lower teeth.*

*Once all of the treatments were complete, he came in for a follow-up beaming from ear to ear. We have before and after pictures of him, side-by-side, and the difference is obvious and remarkable, mostly because of his beaming smile in the "after" picture. At the end of the visit, his wife told me that she can't get him to STOP smiling.*

*Over the course of about a year, I was able to correct his bite, get rid of the clicking, popping, and headaches, as well as fix the chipped and damaged teeth that had caused him so much embarrassment. It was a really enjoyable and satisfying case for me to work on.*

## THE IMPORTANCE OF A PROPER BITE

A large part of the work that I do involves fixing and adjusting the way a patient bites down and the alignment of the jaw when the patient's teeth are closed. The bite I strive to give to all of my patients is one that involves the teeth being properly aligned and the upper and lower jaws and teeth meeting and connecting in a way that is comfortable. The ultimate goal is to have a bite that is stable and that doesn't put excessive strain on the jaw muscles.

It's important that your jaw muscles don't have to do extra work simply to make your teeth come together properly. A proper bite is vitally important: every time we open and close our mouths – which is usually about 3,000 to 5,000 times per day – the jaw muscles fire up. Stress on those muscles can cause pain, sometimes very severe pain, and affect the way you eat, drink, talk, and even sleep.

## UNDERSTANDING YOUR TEMPORAL MANDIBULAR JOINT (TMJ)

The TMJs, right and left, control the movement of your jaw. Problems with your temporal mandibular joint, which are commonly referred to as TMJD – temporal mandibular joint dysfunction – often result from an improper bite, but the dysfunction can also be caused by other things. The bottom line with TMJD is that something in the jaw is not working correctly. In most cases, the dysfunction relates back to an improper bite. A misaligned or improper bite mean that the muscles in the jaw have to work harder to get the teeth to line up and extra stress is put on the TMJs.

If the situation continues untreated, it typically only gets worse. Over time, many patients hear a clicking or popping of the joint, and some patients even experience a locking of the joints, which can prevent them from being able to open or close their mouth.

TMJD can also lead to severe headaches, neck and upper back issues, shoulder problems, dizziness, ringing in the ears, and even vision problems. The muscles of the jaw and face are intimately connected to one another, and when the jaw muscles become overworked, other muscles in the face, head, neck, and shoulders are usually forced to pick up the slack.

## CONTRIBUTING FACTORS AND COMPLICATIONS FROM TMJD

As mentioned earlier, sometimes an incorrect bite isn't the cause of TMJD. In certain cases, a patient's jaw joint simply may not be aligned properly. With some people, the joint has been out of place since birth and never fallen into the right position. They may not even be aware of it until the problem escalates to the point where it causes them noticeable discomfort.

Patients who grind their teeth, or who have had extensive dental work, can also develop a displaced TMJ. There are a variety of different reasons why a patient may have or develop a TMJ that just isn't in the right place, but the end result is inevitably a dysfunctional jaw that causes pain and other problems.

TMJD can cause problems with the teeth themselves. If the jaw muscles are not aligned correctly, and you consistently bite down on your teeth in the wrong position, the teeth can begin to break and chip. I've dealt with a number of patients dealing with TMJD that are incredibly self-conscious about their smile for this reason.

The longer period of time that the TMJ is displaced and that the muscles are strained, the more significant the chipping and breaking becomes. This not only causes patients to be self-conscious about their smile but also affects their basic ability to eat and drink.

Another potential problem is plaque build-up. Trouble with your TMJ can make it painful and even impossible to open your mouth to adequately brush and clean your teeth and mouth. That can easily lead to plaque build-up, decay of the teeth and gums, bad breath, and potentially even infections.

In essence, TMJD is an initial, fundamental problem with a cascading effect, causing multiple other cosmetic and functionality problems.

## Diagnosing TMJD

It's vital to get specifics from a patient, and not all patients present in the same way, but it's generally easy to spot a patient with TMJD. Most TMJD patients have a typical look about them: they generally don't smile much and their faces often have a drawn appearance, tightness around the mouth and cheeks that indicate the strained muscles.

These patients can also develop bagging around the eyes from over-worked facial muscles. Their cheeks may appear enlarged or "chubby" because the overworked jaw joint and muscles can make the cheek areas swell. The forehead usually displays tension or tightness.

The severity of the tightness, strain, and other symptoms is directly related to the type of TMJD the patient has and the length of time they've had it. Still, even patients with an acute TMJD issue – such as a displaced joint due to an accident – frequently display signs of the disorder on their face, and in their neck and shoulders.

## Treating TMJD

One of the first steps to addressing TMJD is to adjust a patient's bite, and the simplest way to do that is with a type of splint. My office uses a specialized computer system to measure muscle activity in the jaw and face. This allows me to determine what muscles are working properly and which muscles are being strained, and that then enables me to design a custom splint to fit the patient's mouth and support the muscles that need it.

The splint sets the bite into the proper position and takes strain off overworked muscles, balancing out the work and keeping the joint from slipping out of alignment.

For this treatment to be effective, it's important that the splint is worn as much as possible. In theory, the splint should be worn 24 hours per day, every single day. However, it's difficult to eat, drink, and effectively brush your teeth and clean your mouth when it's in, so it obviously has to be removed during parts of the day.

Most patients find it difficult to eat with the splint in when they first start wearing it, so, we recommend they remove it for mealtime when necessary, but encourage them to practice wearing the splint during a meal to make the adjustment to eating with the splint in place.

Treating a patient with a splint stops once their muscles and joints have corrected and they can bite and function properly without the splint's correction. The length of time a patient uses a splint depends entirely on them and how long they keep the splint in on a daily basis. I've had some patients that were comfortable after wearing a splint for just a few months.

Other patients have worn a splint for nearly two years before they were comfortable and their jaw was stable without it. It's really a matter of how long it takes for the muscles to begin functioning properly without the splint, and how comfortable the patient is without it.

I generally start out seeing a patient with a splint every few weeks until they start getting comfortable with the splint. After that, a follow-up every four to six weeks is fine, as long as the jaw remains stable. Once the bite is stable, I typically like to address finding a permanent solution or treatment plan – which varies from patient to patient – to prevent their bite and jaw moving back to an improper position.

## TREATMENT COSTS

Cost can be a major deterrent for many patients, but often the long-term health and quality of life costs are far greater. It's hard to put a price tag on the treatment of a patient with TMJD because prices for materials, visits, and specific procedures varies by area and by doctor. Generally speaking, if I treat a patient with a splint and some minor permanent adjustments as a long-term solution, it will usually cost the patient somewhere between $3,000 and $4,000.

If some type of major reconstruction is necessary, or the patient wants or needs major cosmetic adjustments to give them the smile they're looking for, it can cost tens of thousands of dollars. Ultimately, the cost depends on the patient, their individual wants and needs, what type of insurance they have, and what doctor they see for treatment.

Not all insurances will cover treatments – even the treatments used to improve functionality. The primary goal should always be improving functionality, making the jaw as stable and comfortable as possible. Fixing chipped or broken teeth might be part of improving functionality, or it might simply be cosmetic, but that has to be determined on a case-by-case basis.

I want all of my patients to have the best bite and the best smile possible, but, at the end of the day, I want them to be comfortable with the treatment I provide – physically, emotionally, and financially.

## PREVENTING TMJD

Preventing TMJD is a tricky subject because there's no established proven way to accomplish it. The most appropriate solution I've come across is treatment at an early age with functional orthodontics, which is essentially interceptive treatment to ensure that a patient's teeth are developing properly, coming in straight, and that the bite is properly aligned as the patient grows and develops. That's the best way I know of to prevent future TMJD problems, however, it's not foolproof.

Patients with TMJD generally have a lot of questions about the symptoms they're experiencing and the treatment that will be involved to address the symptoms. I encourage my patients to ask questions because it helps them make informed decisions about their care and it usually helps to alleviate any fears or concerns they have.

One of the most common questions I get from patients relates to the treatment they receive and how long the treatment will keep their symptoms at bay. My answer is always the same: I can't guarantee that the treatment I provide will last forever. However, I know from experience that once I've gotten the patient's bite and jaw in the proper position, the treatment will last for as long as the bite and jaw remain in that proper position.

Another common question I get from patients is about orthodontic treatment they received as a child, such as braces, and whether or not that might be the cause of their current bite or jaw problems. I can't say with absolute certainty whether or not a patient's past treatments are the root of their current problems, but in most cases, orthodontic or dental treatments in childhood don't lead to TMJD or bite problems.

In some instances, orthodontic treatment can delay the development of a problem or mask an underlying developmental issue that ultimately causes TMJD in the future. But more often than not, as I noted earlier, orthodontic treatment is usually much more often helpful than harmful.

*One final patient story I'd like to share is about a young woman in her early thirties. She came to see me, complaining of excessive migraine headaches that were drastically affecting her ability to work and to function in any type of social capacity. Her teeth were not chipped or broken, but she'd been grinding them down for a number of years, so much so that each tooth was about half the size it should have been.*

*She avoided smiling because of that wear to her teeth and because of her constant, terrible headaches. She indicated that she often had to leave work and go home to rest because her migraines were so intense. Those headaches were a direct result of her misaligned bite and TMJs resulting from the grinding down of her teeth.*

*From start to finish her case took more than two years to correct. I started her off in a splint to get her comfortable and to help relieve the headaches. The stability of her bite in the splint allowed her muscles to relax, and her headaches became less frequent and less severe.*

*It was then that she mentioned she wanted to improve the look of her smile. In the end, I did a full reconstruction of her teeth, changing each tooth to make it the proper size and color, and making sure that the bite was in the proper position to keep the stress off the joints and the strain off the jaw muscles.*

*She also ended up losing weight and changing other aspects of her physical appearance to accompany her brand new smile. It was a total transformation for her and a huge win for me. Her case reminds me why I do this. I only want the very best for my patients. When they are happy with the end result, I know I've done my job.*

For patients with TMJ issues, it's critically important to find a highly-qualified dentist to provide you with the best possible treatment. I studied at the Las Vegas Institute for Advanced Dental Training, which included a core series of seven different classes. The final step is a fellowship exam which requires the dentist to demonstrate the knowledge gleaned from the classes and how proficient they are with applying the teaching in actually treating patients.

That training was really important, and I've continued to educate myself so that I can feel confident in my abilities to provide all of my patients with the very best possible care.

## ABOUT BRIAN C. MCDOWELL, DDS, LVIF, FIAPA

BrianMcDowellDDS.com

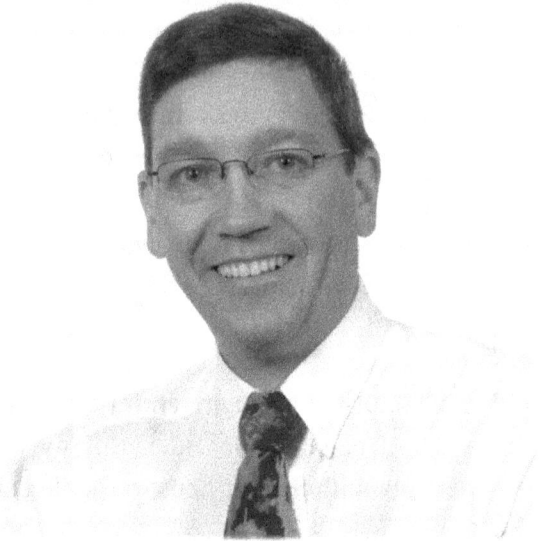

Brian C. McDowell, DDS, is a graduate of the Ohio State University College of Dentistry as well as a Fellow of the prestigious Las Vegas Institute for Advanced Dental Studies. He returned to the Fitchburg/Leominster area in June 1991 after graduating from Ohio State, and in October of that year took over the practice of Dr. Robert Smith in Fitchburg. In 1998, he assumed the practice of Dr. Paul DeLisle and has been at his Electric Avenue location in Fitchburg since that time.

Dr. McDowell is known for his understanding of, and dedication to the personal dental goals of his patients. He and his staff provide the highest quality of care in a relaxed and comfortable atmosphere, with attention to each patient's individual needs. In addition, he and his team attend frequent dental conferences to keep their skills strong in the latest techniques, and Dr. McDowell routinely returns to the Las Vegas Institute for Advanced Dental Studies for training.

Dr. McDowell is an active member of the International Association of Physiologic Aesthetics as well as the American Dental Association, the Massachusetts Dental Society, and the Wachusett District Dental Society, of which he is the current secretary. He also serves as an advisor to the Montachusett Regional Vocation Technical High School Dental Assisting Program and to the Mount Wachusett Community College Dental Hygiene and Dental Assisting Program, helping students acquire the skills that will make them valuable assets to the area's dental profession.

As a Leominster resident, Dr. McDowell understands the local community. He focuses his attention on bringing the best possible dental care to his patients with attention to their personal dental needs. He and his staff provide friendly, professional service to, and evaluate the unique needs of, each patient who visits the practice.

ERNEST MCDOWELL, DMD,
AND RANDY M. FELDMAN, DDS, MS

# LET'S GET SOMETHING STRAIGHT: ORTHODONTICS

Orthodontics is an important aspect of cosmetic dentistry. An orthodontist is a highly-trained specialist who moves teeth to correct misalignment or (malocclusions) improper bites. Having teeth that are properly aligned and fit appropriately are key to overall oral health to having a great smile and enhancing your facial esthetics.

Traditional orthodontic treatment involves the use of braces. Functionally, braces will correct a bite problem resulting from teeth being crooked or otherwise out of proper alignment, and of course, they can also serve the cosmetic purpose of giving you a more attractive smile.

Today, more and more people are very interested in health, in beauty, and their own personal looks. People very much want to look good, feel good and be healthy, and part of that is having perfectly straight teeth for a beautiful "Hollywood smile."

As orthodontists, we want your arches, which means your upper and lower jaw shape, perfectly aligned and fitting together, for comfort, stability, function, health and of course, cosmetic purposes as well.

The braces themselves are actually "small handles" that we glue to the teeth. In the old days, we used metal braces. We advanced later to using ceramic braces. Braces, whether ceramic or metal look like little squares glued on your teeth.

It is the wires that we tie into the braces that supply the force that gets the teeth moving in the desired direction. There are different types of braces, some of which have less friction and move the teeth faster or easier, and there are others that have programmed slots that receive the wires. It used to be the wires that really did all the work. Within the last ten years due to different bracket design and materials the brackets do some of the work as well. With braces the overall process uses varying forces that are delivered through the bracket, the bracket doors (for self-ligating brackets), the wires and the ligation and other auxiliaries utilized.

There are braces that actually self-tie themselves in with doors that hinge closed over the wire, and there are braces that you tie the wire(ligate) in using elastic o-rings. The o-rings come clear, but they also come in a variety of colors, which is something that a lot of kids like.

**Braces for Children**

We generally don't look to do orthodontic treatments before the age of seven. If you start any earlier than that, then there just usually aren't enough permanent teeth present for you to really create any significant improvement. But we do like to see children around that age so that if there are some developing problems, we can catch and treat them early enough to prevent the need for more extensive treatment such as extractions or jaw surgery.

Even though most children do not need treatments then, they should still be screened because you just don't know who does need treatment unless you are able to check them. That's the reason that we (and the AAO) recommend every child be screened early, by age 7.

For patients who do need treatment, we always try to time the start of treatment as efficiently as possible. That way the treatment doesn't take any longer than necessary. With wires that move faster and faster today, if you put braces on too soon, then it doesn't mean that the patient will get the braces off sooner – instead, it just means that they're going to have the braces on for a longer period of time.

## TREATMENT WITH BRACES

As far as how long treatment does take, that can vary widely from one patient to another, depending on the patient's diagnosis, and treatment plan. A number of factors can play into that, such as how much tooth movement required, how much jaw growth or jaw (orthopedic) correction is necessary, just how each patient responds to treatment along with various habits or airway issues. We've had patients that needed as little as three months of orthodontic treatment, and other patients who needed treatment for up to two and a half years.

The required treatment time can also vary depending on what the patient's expressed desires are about what they would like us to do for them. A simple one tooth cross bite may take a lot less time than treatment designed to achieve an overall comprehensive result that includes not only great function but also ideal cosmetic results. This latter scenario usually includes precise tooth measurements and the collaboration of an excellent cosmetic dentist and periodontist as well. In this manner, the shape, size, position, emergence profile, incisal display, gingival relation, lip fullness and relation are all recognized, diagnosed and intimately addressed!

The necessary frequency of office visits during treatment is also something that varies from patient to patient, depending on the nature of the treatment and how the individual patient responds. If we're doing orthopedic treatment on the jaw, office visits may vary greatly.

When talking about (dentofacial) orthopedic treatment, there are cases where we may need to develop a patient's upper and lower jaws a bit more to create sufficient space so that there's a better chance of avoiding adult teeth extractions later.

It is very important to treat children while they're young and still growing, dentofacial orthopedic work on the jaws is very important in preventing more invasive procedures later.

We can widen jaws with orthopedic movements. We can also maximize the jaw's genetic growth potential by placing the jaws in certain positions that stimulate jaw growth. There are now special appliances that we can have custom fabricated which attach to the teeth and will begin to either expand or advance the jaws in certain positions that stimulate muscle and bone growth, thereby obviating any orthopedic disharmony resulting in a great profile without surgery! A BIG WIN!

By working both on the position and shape of the jaws, along with straightening the patient's teeth, we can dramatically improve someone's appearance, and the overall look of their face.

Facial appearance shows improvement, also their profile, and at the same time the alignment of their teeth.

For general orthodontic treatment with braces, we typically only need to see patients about once every eight to ten weeks. We don't usually need to see patients with braces as often as we did in the past, thanks to developing more advanced wires that keep the teeth moving over a longer time without needing adjustments. That's really an important advance because it means patients don't have to come in as often and miss work or school as often as was the case in the past. Additionally, there is MUCH less discomfort with the newer futuristic wires.

We do want to also check patients regularly to see if they're having any particular problems with discomfort. Some patients are apprehensive about pain or discomfort from wearing braces. We try to allay those concerns by using the analogy of having a bruise. It's sort of like having a bruise on your arm. It doesn't hurt all the time, but if you press on it, it definitely feels tender or sore. In the same way, when you put pressure on your teeth by biting, especially right after having your braces tightened up, then you're going to feel some soreness.

But it's not like walking around with a severe toothache all day. It's just the normal inflammatory and healing response that comes from the fact that we are gradually moving the actual roots of the teeth through the jaw bone.

## MAINTENANCE OF BRACES

We recommend patients keep their braces clean through normal, good oral hygiene using a toothbrush, toothpaste, flossing, electric toothbrushes, or a Waterpik or similar device.

With children, we tell parents to basically use anything that will help motivate your child to keep their teeth clean. Simple frequent brushing and flossing are just as good as anything as long as they're done properly. We do spend a lot of time teaching and educating patients about how to take care of their teeth.

We also recommend prescription strength fluoride rinse to keep the enamel hard and resistant to cavities. Other than that, just brushing with regular toothpaste with fluoride works great.

## BRACES FOR ADULTS

Braces are beneficial for just about anyone in terms of improving both their bite and their appearance. About the only person we would hesitate to put braces on would be patient's with periodontal(gum) disease that renders the underlying bone not healthy enough to support movement of the teeth.

Approximately 40% of our practice consists of treating adults. A lot of that is treatment with braces, but a lot more adults are now choosing clear aligner therapy such as Invisalign. Our practice, Blue Wave Orthodontics is in the Top 1% of Invisalign providers Worldwide, and that has substantially increased the number of adults we treat.

Within the past 15 years we have definitely seen a significant increase in the number of adults seeking orthodontic treatment. It's just become more and more socially desirable to have a really nice, attractive smile. That's usually the first thing someone notices when they look at you for the first time.

Over time, the stigma of having braces has been far outweighed by the stigma of not having a beautiful, straight smile. That's one reason more and more adults are getting treatment. We think the choice of having clear braces, replacing the metal braces that we used to use, has led to more people seeking out orthodontic cosmetic treatment. Plus, treatment times are faster now than before, because of the high-tech wires and brackets that we have available now, that move the teeth faster.

We do have to do some combination orthodontic treatment because sometimes, with some tooth movements, braces and wires will fix better, and some things aligners such as Invisalign will fix better. So, once in a while we may do some certain movements with braces and then complete the treatment with Invisalign. That way, instead of the patient having to have braces on for a year and a half to two years, they may only have braces on for three or four months, and then we can move them to treatment with Invisalign and finish in another 8-10 months.

## THE DEVELOPMENT OF ALIGNERS

Treatment with aligners began in 1999. The new concept developed uses a succession, or progression, of clear aligners – aligners are essentially like clear retainers – that incrementally move your teeth more gently and easily without having to use braces. Invisalign is the main and original system developed. There are other aligner systems out there now, such as Clear Correct, but Invisalign still holds the original patent on the technology and is the aligner treatment of choice.

With Invisalign, you can go to an orthodontist, and they will scan your teeth with an optical/digital scanner to create an image. It takes about three minutes to take an image of the upper arch, and another three minutes to take an image of the lower arch.

Working on a computer from that image, sort of like working with a CAD – computer assisted design – program, the orthodontist is able to create a progressive series of clear trays called aligners to quickly move your teeth. This enables them to be incredibly precise, by modeling each tray based on the most recent scan, so that the orthodontist can create for the patient exactly the look, bite and smile that is desired.

Because the aligner trays are clear, there's no embarrassment for the patient in the way there once was with metal braces.

## TREATMENT WITH INVISALIGN

Invisalign is a huge technological advance and quite frankly the first MAJOR paradigm shift to treat malocclusions since the specialty began in 1901. Invisalign enables us to treat patients over the age of 12 - basically anyone who has all their permanent teeth in – and get amazing results usually within a treatment time of just 12 months. Invisalign has enabled us to get great cosmetic results, often without doing extractions or surgery.

Treating the average patient with Invisalign takes about 12 months. The orthodontist uses an average of 48 lower and upper aligner models, designed from the 3D image scans. A UV light polymerizing resin is the main ingredient of the model, so we can take the Invisalign material and process it on each incrementally varied resin model. The "Smart Track" Align material is pressed down on the model, and a robotics program guides a laser to cut it. The freshly formed aligners are now tumbled with a bunch of ceramic beads to smooth the edges. They are then computer assisted labeled and bagged.

So now you have 48 sets of incrementally progressive aligners. The patient wears each set 22 hours a day for a week (or two) and then goes on to the next one. The aligners progressively move your teeth and you get a wonderful result at the end.

When the Invisalign treatment is complete, some patients may need some refinement, just tweaking the results a bit to get things even more ideal. The orthodontist does another scan and creates an additional three or four months' worth of trays that the patient wears to get really perfect results if needed or desired.

Also, patients will wear a retainer at night after completing the Invisalign treatment, to hold their results! Many opt for the Invisalign retainer called Vivera which is made like the aligners that move your teeth, only with Vivera they hold the final position!

And "voila", you are done and have gorgeous results with "look Ma, NO braces"!

Invisalign is an amazing technology, a total paradigm shift. It's almost like if you wanted to travel from New York to Los Angeles and the only available travel choices were train, bus, or car. In regard to orthodontics, Invisalign is like the paradigm shift that occurred when suddenly people were able to travel by airplane!

## ADVANTAGES OF ALIGNERS

Probably about 95% of our adult patients use Invisalign. The only situations where we wouldn't use Invisalign are if the patient has an impacted tooth – a tooth stuck in their gums – or some other situation that necessitates surgery.

Some patients may need periodontal work done before they can use Invisalign. If you're going to move teeth, you've got to have a good, solid foundation for the teeth. You can't move teeth if the patient has significant periodontal or gum disease because there's not a strong enough foundation. Those patients would first need treatment by a periodontist who examines them to decide which teeth are good and which ones are poor or guarded. We would remove the poor teeth and the guarded ones need cleaning before you can do orthodontic treatment.

Aligners can offer several advantages over using braces. Braces can stick to your teeth and bother your lips. Also, braces can potentially damage the enamel coating on the teeth, especially with poor oral hygiene. Although that's not as big a problem now as it was when braces were always made of metal. Braces can pick up a little food debris where the bracket meets the tooth, and then bacteria can begin to cause decay.

What can happen if the patient doesn't brush well enough and the dentist doesn't catch it, when they take off the brackets, there are little white rings on their teeth, the beginnings of a cavity AKA decalcification. Potentially, that might mean having to get bonding or veneers after straightening the teeth. When you use aligner therapy, you don't have that problem.

With braces, you also still have the social stigma of wearing them, which bothers some patients, and more pain or discomfort than you have with aligners.

With Invisalign, you can just pop the aligners on and off, take them off for eating or for a date or other social engagement. They feel much more comfortable than braces, and they don't affect your speech. Plus, you don't have the problem that braces have of picking up plaque and bacteria. With aligners, you're changing the tray every week or two, so you regularly have a brand-new tray that's fresh and clean.

Having recommended aligners from the beginning, since 1999 we have had many celebrities, beauty contestants, sports figures, musician, weather announcers and news broadcasters that wear them as prescribed, i.e. all the time, when performing and "on the air" with no issues at all!

Aligners are clean, they're healthy, and they look good. Most people cannot even tell when you have a clear aligner on. That's one of the reasons that so many adults absolutely love Invisalign treatment, because it doesn't show like braces do.

## COST OF ORTHODONTIC TREATMENTS

As a general rule, the cost for treatment with braces ranges from about $3,000 to around $7,000, depending upon the type and length of treatment and what part of the world you live in. Patients who finance the treatment typically pay about $150 to $250 per month in payments, depending upon the dental practice's financing policies. Many practices, including ours, offer an in-house financing plan.

Dental insurance, depending on the company, usually covers part of the cost, but usually not all of it, which is why most orthodontists offer patients a financing or payment plan.

Aligners, depending upon the length of treatment, run in about the same price range, from around $3,000 up to about $7,500.

Our practice is Invisalign/Braces neutral, meaning we charge the same to get the malocclusion corrected. We do NOT surcharge for Invisalign.

The generally reduced orthodontic treatment times have made it easier for dentists to offer their patients financing, since obviously, the cost depends a lot on how many times, and for how long overall we need to see and treat the patient.

## EFFECTIVENESS OF ORTHODONTIC TREATMENTS

Orthodontics treatments are really one of the most effective cosmetic dental procedures. They can make a big difference in someone's life. We get a lot of satisfaction when we can do something like treat a child who's been teased about the appearance of their teeth, and watch the treatment help them blossom into an outgoing, self-confident kid. That's one of the most rewarding parts of our profession.

We also treat a lot of adults that choose to finally get their teeth fixed, and the most common thing they say is that they wish they'd done it sooner. Just like with treating children, we've treated a lot of adults and have satisfaction seeing how getting their teeth fixed with braces or aligners just completely changes their personality as far as their self-esteem, self-confidence, and just their overall satisfaction in life.

Most HR people involved with interviewing job candidates always note one's smile is the most significant part of the non-verbal interview, and that makes all the difference.

Here's the story of just one case we treated. *The patient was a female air force officer in her late 20s. She had what's referred to as a severe Class III – that's where the lower jaw is much more forward than the upper jaw. She also had a severe underbite, the lower front teeth being way out in the front of the upper front teeth.*

*She could have easily been a candidate for jaw surgery, but she specifically said that she didn't want to have jaw surgery.*

*We decided to go with Invisalign, which we thought we could make work for her without needing surgery. We had to extract her two lower front teeth, but after 15 months of Invisalign treatment, we had closed up that space where the two teeth were removed, her underbite vanished and we were basically able to get the same results as if she'd had jaw surgery.*

*She was absolutely thrilled, both with the awesome results we were able to get for her and for the fact that she didn't have to have jaw surgery. Her "before" and "after" pictures show just an amazing transformation in her looks, and she, herself, said that the Invisalign treatment changed her life.*

The technological advances that we've made in orthodontics, the development of better braces and the introduction of the Invisalign technology, have made it much easier for both children and adults to get fantastic results as far as transforming their smile into a real work of art. We urge anyone who has a problem with the alignment of their teeth or their bite to look into their options by seeing and talking with an orthodontist.

## ABOUT RANDY M. FELDMAN, DDS, MS & ERNEST MCDOWELL, DMD

Blue Wave Orthodontics
BluewaveOrtho.com

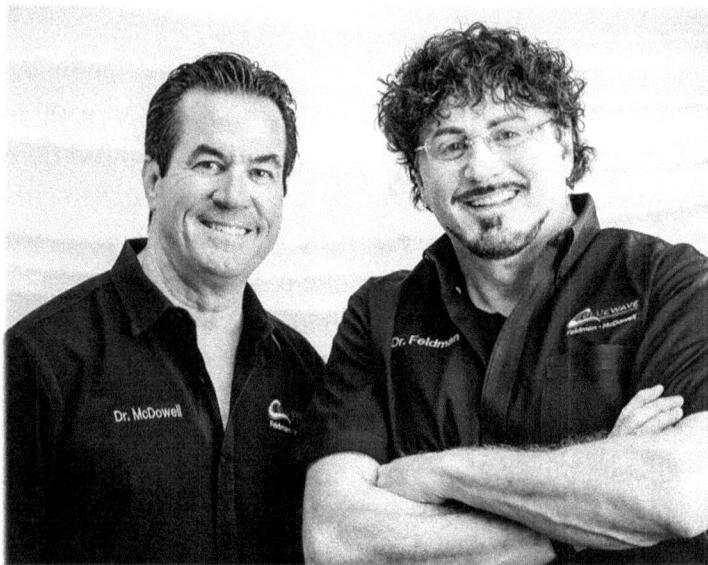

Dr. Randy Feldman and Dr. Ernest McDowell have spent many years helping patients obtain beautiful, healthy smiles. As trusted orthodontists with years of experience, they work diligently to ensure that every patient receives the best possible care and smiles that boost self-confidence.

Dr. Randy Feldman received his BA in zoology from The Ohio State University, where he also obtained his DDS and MS in orthodontics. He is a Clinical Associate Professor in the Department of Pediatrics at USF College of Medicine. He also holds a patent for one of his contributions to the dental field, ceramic brackets. His passion is pediatric orthodontics, and for more than 30 years, he has been helping children obtain the smiles that they deserve. His special focus is helping special needs children. He is the former President of the Make-A-Wish

Foundation, sits on the board of directors for Voices for Children, and serves as a Guardian Ad Litem to the Florida judicial system. He is also the President of More Health, Inc., a group that promotes health education for students in Pinellas and Hillsborough Counties, and established the Feldman Orthodontics Scholarship Program to help send local Bay area students to college.

Additionally, Dr. Feldman is an early adopter of the Invisalign technique (1999) and is not only in the Top 1% of providers Worldwide, but he has also treated over 3,000 patients with this new innovative orthodontic process.

Dr. Feldman is a member of the American Association of Orthodontics, American College of Dentists (Fellow), American Cleft Palate Association, American Orthodontic Society, International College of Orthodontists (Fellow), American Dental Association, Southeastern Society of Pediatric Dentistry, Southern Association of Orthodontists, Florida Dental Association, Hillsborough County Dental Association (Past President), Tampa Bay Academy of General Dentistry (Mastership) and Schulman Study Group, as well as many other professional and community organizations. A few of his awards include the Tampa Bay Business Journal Health Care Hero, Greater Tampa Chamber Business of the Year (1997), Lifetime Achievement Award by the Hillsborough County Dental Association in 2011 and chosen as the Tampa Bay Lightning Community Hero in 2015.

Dr. Ernest H. McDowell has been working with patients to create beautiful smiles since 1987. As a board-certified orthodontist, he is a member of an elite group of professionals. He focuses on cutting-edge techniques that help him diagnose and treat all types of malocclusions. He has been awarded the Elite

Provider Status for Invisalign due to his extensive level of education and experience, an honor bestowed upon only one percent of Invisalign Providers across the globe.

Born and raised in Pinellas County, Dr. McDowell is a 1977 graduate of Dixie Hollins High School. He received his BA in Biology from the University of South Florida and his D.M.D. degree from the University of Florida, where he graduated with honors in 1985. He completed a residency in Orthodontics at the University of Louisville in 1987, then returned to practice in Pinellas County. He lectures at both the University of Florida and Nova University, and has been published in national orthodontics publications. He also presents regularly on orthodontic topics in both national and international venues. He was president of the Upper Pinellas Dental Board in 2003.

Dr. McDowell stays active in his community, sponsoring Little League and softball teams throughout Pinellas County, as well as local health fairs, YMCA events, and community projects.

Both Dr. Feldman and Dr. McDowell are committed to providing patients with compassionate, professional dental care.

# THE CONSEQUENCES OF MISSING TEETH

According to the latest statistics about 35 million Americans don't have any teeth and around 178 million Americans are missing at least one tooth. If that is not alarming enough, those numbers are projected to increase over the next two decades.

Missing teeth, if not restored by good dental treatment, lead to an ever-increasing number of severe problems. Missing teeth affect your appearance, the bone structure of your face, and the total health of your body.

If you lose a tooth, it's important to take action to get dental restoration as soon as possible. Taking prompt action will reduce the cost and, more importantly, will prevent a chain reaction of potential negative consequences from occurring.

## THE CAUSES OF MISSING TEETH

One of the main reasons that people lose teeth is simply a lack of understanding how our mouth works. The average person will only go to a dentist when a problem gets to the point where it's causing them pain. That is a wrong-headed approach. The fact is that most of the things that can go wrong in our mouth do not hurt us at all. They don't provide pain as a warning sign. Pain is more often a sign that substantial damage has already occurred.

By the time a person experiences pain from a dental problem, it's usually too late in the sense that it will take an expensive procedure like a root canal and crown to repair the damage.

I think we need to do a better job of communicating to people the importance of regular dental visits. Regular visits are vital to their health, regardless of whether you feel like you have a problem. A dentist can spot problems long before the point of causing pain or significantly damaging the teeth or gums.

Periodontal disease and bacteria are the main immediate causes of tooth loss. Again, these are problems that a dentist can spot very early on and easily and successfully treat before the problem gets anywhere near losing a tooth. But the average person is not going to notice a problem with periodontal disease until it's very advanced and has already done substantial damage.

There are about eight billion bacteria in our mouth all the time, producing acids and toxins that can potentially infect the gums. When infected, gum tissue becomes inflamed and pulls away from the teeth and from the bacteria. Then the infection goes on to affect the bone substructure beneath the gums, and before you know it, the gum and the bone are pulling away from the bacteria. Still, a person isn't likely to experience a lot of pain until the teeth are already loose from infection.

Periodontal disease is the number one cause of tooth loss. Besides that, there are various sorts of trauma such as car accidents or sports injuries that cause tooth loss. People can't do anything beforehand to prevent trauma injuries but they can prevent periodontal disease by practicing good oral hygiene and seeing a dentist regularly, at least once a year if not every six months. Once every six months is ideal.

## EFFECTS OF MISSING TEETH - APPEARANCE AND ATTITUDE

Most people are significantly affected in a personal way by missing teeth. The effects range from concerns about their appearance to having severe issues with self-confidence or self-esteem. If you're missing a tooth, especially one of your front teeth, you know that people notice it.

Your smile is very important. It's one of the most important aspects of how people perceive you when they first meet you. If your smile is less than perfect, people notice.

In my practice, I try to help each person and I want to make sure that I meet the individual needs and desires of each patient. There are many issues involved with missing teeth. I don't preach to my patients, "You've got a missing tooth and this is going to cause you issues." I prefer to let patients tell me what issues bother them.

Honestly, anyone would be concerned about a missing tooth right up front, about the aesthetics and how it looks. It's been my experience with patients that if it affects your appearance that much, it is also going to have a substantial negative effect on your psychological health. Common statements or questions that I hear from patients, that indicate their concerns, are things like, "I feel like I can't talk to people. I can't smile. How can I go to work? I'm not comfortable being out in public or with a group of people."

When people are missing teeth, typically the first thing to happen is that they stop smiling. Feeling embarrassed is a very common reaction. You're not comfortable in social situations. Your confidence and self-esteem go down.

Ultimately, missing teeth can significantly impact all of your relationships, personal, social, or business relationships, in a negative way. When you're feeling embarrassed and reluctant to smile, you tend to back away from all interactions with people, and that will basically affect your whole life.

I've had patients who were mothers that even became reluctant to smile at their children. That's a terrible situation and one that makes someone feel just absolutely awful. When you're a parent and you can't smile in front of your children, not only does it affect your life, it also affects your children's lives. When a patient tells me something like that, it's nothing short of heart-wrenching.

*Like a patient I had not long ago – a mother who was missing a tooth, and it got to the point where she hardly ever smiled. She knew that was a bad example for her children, and that was one of the driving factors that prompted her to want to get the tooth replaced.*

*Once I replaced that tooth she smiled in front of her kids with tears in her eyes when she saw the restoration. Honestly, I had tears in my eyes, too. That was a big deal for me to be able to do that for her as a dentist.*

These are the issues that we see with missing teeth. Teeth are a natural part of the body. When you look at someone, you expect to see two arms, two legs, two eyes… and a smile. If that smile is missing, it's going to draw attention, negative attention.

## EFFECTS OF MISSING TEETH — BITE SHIFT

A very significant practical effect of missing teeth is bite shift and misalignment.

A lot of people don't understand the tremendous wear and tear that teeth suffer. The mouth is a very harsh environment. When the average person bites down while chewing food, they're putting pressure on their teeth equal to approximately twice their body weight.

That's a tremendous amount of pressure. Think about how many times a day, every day, that pressure is applied. When you realize that, it's really no surprise that over time our teeth can wear out.

When you bite down, the pressure from your bite is usually carried slightly forward, so the pressure is going toward the front of the mouth. The first molars are usually the first teeth that many people have problems with or lose, because they take a lot of that pressure since they're primary teeth used in chewing our food. They're the first "extra" teeth to come in when we lose our baby teeth and start getting our adult, permanent teeth.

If a person loses that first molar tooth, then the overall forward pressure on teeth causes the second molar, the tooth immediately behind it, to begin to collapse forward into the space that's left. Also, if you lose a first molar on the bottom, then the tooth above it is going to drop down. However, if you lose an upper first molar, then the tooth below it is going to start to rise up out of the gum.

Teeth will always tend to move forward and they'll always be erupting. The lower teeth are going to erupt up and the top teeth are going to erupt down until they meet resistance. That's how your bite starts to get out of a proper, straight, firm alignment.

I often compare the mouth to a stone-arched bridge. If you have an arched bridge made of stones and one of those stones falls out, then the bridge is going to begin to collapse because the other stones will no longer be held firmly in place. It works the same way with your teeth.

Once you lose one tooth, the pressures that move the remaining teeth can cause a chain reaction of problems that can cause you to lose more teeth. If you lose your first molar, then as pressure causes the second molar to lean forward into that space, more pressure is applied to the back part of the second molar and then that tooth starts to get loose.

That potential chain reaction effect that threatens other teeth is one reason that I strongly urge patients to replace a missing tooth as quickly as possible.

Teeth shift very easily. That's how orthodontics – braces, for example – work, by moving your teeth. It doesn't take a lot of force to move teeth. Even very slight but constant force will do the trick. Our tongue can move teeth. Children that have a thumb-sucking habit will make the front teeth begin to grow sticking out, just from that slight pressure. Teeth will move very easily by pressure, whether it's from the tongue, the cheeks, braces, or as a result of missing teeth.

When the teeth begin to shift because of a missing tooth, that messes up your bite alignment because the teeth are not sitting properly. Without that missing tooth, the teeth are going to move into a position that is not in proper alignment, and that's going to lead to further breakdown.

Think of the door on a very old car. You lift the door handle and you can feel the door moving a bit. It's loose. Maybe it makes a harsh squeaking sound. It doesn't open smoothly because it's not tightly in the proper place. It's gotten out of line. It's kind of like that when your teeth move out of proper alignment.

Our mouth should be able to open and close smoothly, and our teeth need to be in proper alignment with one another for chewing. A missing tooth causes the remaining teeth to shift to places they shouldn't. That puts excessive and unbalanced force on our bite, and also on our jaw joints.

That's how people get breakdown of the temporomandibular joint (TMJ), the hinge that connects the jaw to the temporal bones of your skull. That can lead to jaw pain, headaches, a whole host of problems.

As I said, having a tooth missing just starts a chain reaction that continues to cause one problem after another. By saying that, I'm referring to problems with your teeth, your jaw - which affects your facial appearance, and also to problems with your overall physical health.

## EFFECTS OF MISSING TEETH – DIGESTION AND HEALTH ISSUES

There are consequences of missing teeth that people don't usually think about, consequences related to your overall health. The mouth is the pathway to your body for all the nutrients it needs. Our teeth, giving us the ability to chew food, is part of the process our body needs to take in those necessary nutrients. If we can't chew our food correctly, then we can't digest our food correctly.

Without the proper teeth in the proper place and position, you can't chew your food correctly. You're going to end up swallowing larger chunks of food that haven't been adequately chewed and that, therefore, your body can't digest properly. Not being able to digest your food properly can lead to intestinal problems, obesity, malnutrition, and illness.

One problem that develops, a problem that can directly lead to malnutrition and poor overall health, is that people with missing teeth often avoid eating certain foods that are harder to chew but that are very important to our health. Instead, they start to favor eating less healthy foods, such as candy bars or other "junk food", that are easier to chew.

## EFFECTS OF MISSING TEETH — BONE LOSS

Bone loss in the jaw is a major problem that results from missing teeth. Our jaws are very unique bones in our body. There's no other bone in your body that if you don't use it, it begins to go away. However, if a tooth is missing, our body will actually tend to take away bone from our jawbones.

Over time, you can lose a very significant amount of bone in your jaw, which is, of course, the structure that supports your teeth and your whole face.

Sometimes, if someone loses a tooth in the back, they tend to think, "Well, nobody sees that so I'm not going to worry about getting it replaced". What they don't understand is that the missing tooth leads to bone loss in the jaw. Then that bone loss increases tooth alignment problems, which then leads to further dental and health problems.

Just because people can't see a missing tooth right away, that doesn't mean that missing tooth isn't causing you any problems.

As time passes, if you don't have a missing tooth restored right away, the resulting bone loss also makes it difficult to repair the missing tooth because it can get to the point where the bone has eroded so much that it can't hold a dental implant, which is the preferred dental restoration treatment for a missing tooth.

If someone gets an implant to replace a missing tooth right away, that's usually a pretty easy procedure, and the implant tooth replacement will prevent further bone loss from happening. But if someone waits several years after losing a tooth before trying to get it fixed, restored, then they may need bone grafting surgery to even be able to get a dental implant.

If a person loses multiple teeth and doesn't do anything about it, then the bone loss is going to accelerate, more bone will be lost faster, and that can make it difficult for a person to even use the less than ideal option of getting dentures. It will be difficult to fit dentures properly; they'll have to replace the dentures more often; it will also be more difficult to hold the dentures firmly in place. The patient will be more prone to experience dentures falling out or breaking.

Bone loss also causes significant problems with your facial appearance. It causes your cheeks to sag and it causes wrinkles. The whole shape of your face changes over time. Your jaw line and the shape of your face will narrow. Basically, it will make you look a lot older than you actually are. That gets back to the cosmetic issues that I talked about earlier.

## SOLUTIONS FOR MISSING TEETH — DOING NOTHING

There are several dental treatment options for dealing with missing teeth. I don't tell patients what to do. I give them choices. Ultimately, it is the patient's decision because it's the patient's body.

One choice, of course, is to do nothing, to just have a missing tooth and not do anything about it as far as getting a dental restoration. I don't think that's ever a good option, but it is an option, and so I present it as an option when I talk with patients, explaining the relative advantages and disadvantages just as I do with any other option.

The only advantages to doing nothing are not having to take the time to go to the dentist for treatment and not spending the money for the cost of a restoration. But even those aren't really advantages, or they're just short-term advantages because choosing not to take care of a missing tooth now just means that eventually you will suffer more severe dental problems that you'll have to take care of later. That's probably going to mean even more trips to the dentist and spending more money than if you'd taken care of your missing tooth problem right away.

Other possible disadvantages of doing nothing include all the consequences of missing teeth that I've already mentioned: embarrassment, loss of self-confidence and self-esteem, relationship problems, and all the practical dental and other health issues such as bite shift, malnutrition, intestinal problems, and bone loss.

## SOLUTIONS FOR MISSING TEETH — DENTURES

One choice of treatment is a removable dental appliance, either partial or whole dentures. Dentures offer the advantage of being a lower cost, more affordable option. Dentures can solve cosmetic appearance and bite alignment problems, but they don't solve the problem of bone loss.

That's why people with dentures usually have to get a new denture made every few years. The ongoing, gradual bone loss causes their jaw to shrink, and eventually it gets to the point where their dentures don't fit any longer and they need new denture plates. .

Some patients just aren't comfortable with dentures because the dentures can move around in their mouth. Dentures aren't firmly attached in the way that a crown, a bridge, or an implant is. They can even fall out, right when you're in the middle of eating, talking, or laughing. That causes some patients a lot of anxiety because they're worried about the potential embarrassment of having their denture pop out in front of people.

One thing that can significantly improve using dentures as a treatment option is getting an implant-supported denture. That's a treatment procedure that was just developed in the past several years. The procedure involves an implant – surgically attaching an artificial, metal root to the jawbone - and then attaching the denture to the implant.

The implant obviously is going to hold a denture in place much more firmly than the way dentures are typically held in place just by suction or with an adhesive. Using an implant-supported denture can help avoid problems such as gum irritation or gum sores that are usually caused by loose dentures wearing on the gums.

## SOLUTIONS FOR MISSING TEETH – BRIDGE RESTORATIONS

Bridges are a better option than dentures. A bridge is a fixed dental restoration, not something that you take out – or that can fall out or get lost. A dental bridge is more effective as a tooth replacement because it effectively prevents that potential chain reaction of your bite getting out of alignment after you lose a tooth. It accomplishes that by attaching an artificial tooth to two adjacent, existing teeth.

A dental bridge can provide an excellent cosmetic restoration of your smile and can enable you to function normally in terms of eating, smiling, and talking. However, a bridge restoration, while it will help to slow down bone loss in the jaw, won't completely stop bone loss from occurring.

## SOLUTIONS FOR MISSING TEETH – DENTAL IMPLANTS

What I consider the ideal solution for a missing tooth is a dental implant, a procedure that replaces a whole tooth, both the root part of the tooth as well as the visible top part of the tooth. The dentist implants an artificial root in the jawbone where the missing tooth root was located and then places a crown on top of that.

Dental implants offer a number of advantages over a bridge. A key advantage of a dental implant is that since it directly replaces the original root of a tooth in the jawbone, it prevents further bone loss. It stabilizes the adjoining teeth and your bite alignment, and it also provides a really beautiful cosmetic solution that restores your smile.

Of all the possible treatment options, an implant is the only one that's going to work perfectly to prevent bone loss. With a bridge, you're still going to get some bone loss over time.

Also, implants are easier to clean and maintain than a bridge that can sometimes get food particles underneath the artificial tooth in a bridge.

Another advantage with an implant you don't have to do anything to other, healthy teeth. With a bridge, you have to take some of the enamel off of the teeth that anchor the bridge – that the bridge is attached to – and crown those teeth, even if the teeth are perfectly healthy.

What the patient can afford is also a factor that needs to be considered. Obviously, if you need bone augmentation surgery then that's going to be a lot more expensive than just getting a simple implant.

As a doctor, I always want to make sure that I fully inform my patient of all their possible options, even though I generally consider a dental implant to be the best option. The patient, not the dentist, should ultimately decide. My job is to educate patients on the pros and cons, advantages and disadvantages, of each option that's available to them, so that they have all the information they need to make a wise, informed choice.

## MISSING TEETH — HOW TO AVOID TOOTH LOSS

I've talked a lot about problems and solutions concerning missing teeth, but I want to make sure that people understand how important regular dental checkups and cleanings are to prevent this from happening in the first place.

One analogy that I find often helps patients to clearly understand the importance of regular dental visits is that of owning a nice, expensive automobile. Now, if all you ever do is just put gas in the car and drive it around, but you fail to do regular maintenance on the car, well, eventually that car is going to break down.

It's like that with your teeth, too. If you don't go in for regular maintenance on them, eventually they're going to start breaking down. In the same way that your car won't necessarily show any noticeable problems when it's time for an oil change, your teeth may not hurt or cause you any obvious problems when it's time for a once-every-six-months dental visit. You still need to go in for that dental visit though, just like you need to take your car in for an oil change.

If you keep driving your car without changing the oil, at some point the car will break down and stop working altogether. Failing to provide proper maintenance for your teeth will work the same way. It will end up resulting in a severe breakdown that will be more expensive to repair than what regular maintenance cost.

## THE DIFFERENCE REPLACING A MISSING TOOTH CAN MAKE IN YOUR LIFE

I also want people to understand the tremendous benefits they can experience from properly replacing a missing tooth. I have a lot of wonderful stories about the results of someone taking proper action to replace missing teeth.

*I remember one patient that I had several years ago, a young lady in her 20s. When she came to see me she had a lot of dental issues so she saved her money for restoration. She had several missing teeth and, like most people, she was very self-conscious and embarrassed. She was very quiet and came off as appearing very shy and reserved. She didn't smile much, or even talk very much, because she was so self-conscious of her mouth and the appearance of her teeth.*

*I did a lot of crown and bridgework to replace her missing teeth and to restore a really beautiful smile for her. It took a while to do all the necessary work, but as we were doing it, I could see all these wonderful changes unfolding in her personality. She grew her hair out a bit. She started dressing better, dressing up more – trading in jeans with holes in them for nice skirts and dresses. And of course she started to smile again.*

*She underwent a very noticeable and wonderfully attractive transformation, not just in her appearance but also in her attitude. Her self-esteem, her confidence, the way she interacted with people – all of those things dramatically improved. She became a lot more relaxed, a lot more outgoing, and a lot more comfortable and at ease in social situations.*

*During the time we were working on her – a period of about six to seven months – as her self-confidence improved, she was able to go out and get a better job. She just had a better life overall because she felt so much better about herself. Once she was able to smile, she was able to relax and let herself go. You could see her personality beginning to shine through. Having her missing teeth fixed completely changed her life.*

Your teeth are important, and not just for chewing, but also for your entire existence. Your smile is important. It's one of the first things that people notice about you, and it's one of the features of your face that makes the strongest first impression.

Make the small efforts necessary to take good care of your teeth – brushing and flossing, and regular visits to a dentist. And if you do lose a tooth, either from tooth decay or from an injury, go talk with your dentist about it right away and discuss your treatment options and make the best treatment choice for yourself. Choosing any treatment is going to be a much better solution than doing nothing. And you'll probably be very pleasantly surprised by what a big difference getting a missing tooth replaced makes in your life.

# About Stephen DeLoach, DDS

Center for Dental Excellence
DicksonDentist.com

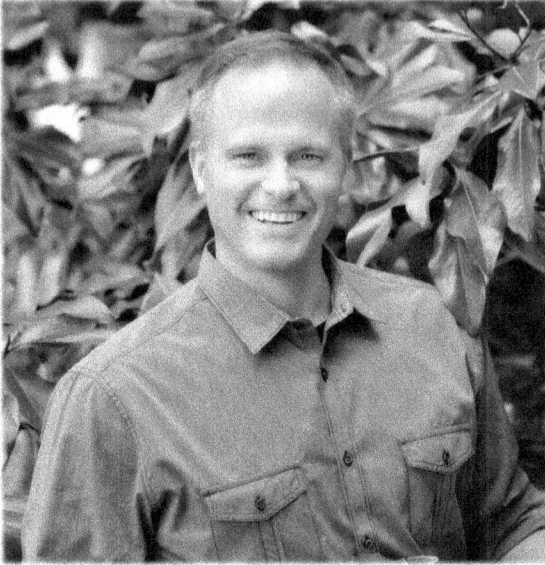

When Dr. Stephen DeLoach began practicing dentistry, he had two goals in mind. First, he wanted to exhibit the very best in dental care and technology from around the world. Second, he wanted to deliver a very special brand of care for his patients in a comfortable setting that would uphold the core values of family and community that meant so much to him. Today, Dr. DeLoach and his team are living this dream by providing superior dental services to the Dickson area.

Upon graduation from the University of Tennessee School of Dentistry, Dr. DeLoach began to achieve this dream by traveling to the Dawson Center for Advanced Dental Study in Tampa, Florida. There, he learned more about how to help those who are suffering from head, neck and jaw joint pain. He also traveled to the Las Vegas Institute for Advanced Dental Studies, where he learned to incorporate modern laser techniques as well as other technologies into his daily practice. Finally, he went to Boston, where he attended a symposium on cosmetic dentistry that drew professionals from all over the world to share their knowledge and skill.

Now, Dr. DeLoach is bringing these years of study back to his hometown area. Incorporating the skills he has learned through his years of practice, he and his staff offer compassionate and professional dental service to patients in Dickson, including implant dentistry and other cosmetic procedures. Dr. DeLoach and his staff also offer preventative dentistry services such as professional cleaning and sedation dentistry, for those who may need it.

As part of his efforts to deliver professional care to patients in the Dickson area, Dr. DeLoach, along with his trained and friendly staff, offer the best in dental treatment with a hometown approach so that patients are always comfortable.

# FILLING-IN THE GAPS WITH BRIDGES AND DENTURES

Two important dental treatments that serve both functional, or restorative, and cosmetic purposes for patients are dentures and bridges. Approximately 15% of the U.S. population use dentures, and more than half of the population is missing at least one tooth.

Bridges or dentures can be used to replace lost teeth and to improve the appearance of your smile. *One example comes from a young lady I had as a patient, who was playing basketball, got elbowed and had her front teeth knocked out when she was only 19 years old. She wore a denture for a while, but she wasn't really happy with it – she was very self-conscious about how she looked, was worried about her smile, and just didn't like wearing the denture.*

*She decided to that the denture wasn't the restoration that she wanted. When she visited my office, I went through the various options with her, including dental implants, and ended up replacing her missing teeth with a bridge because she did not want to wait the time that it would take to complete the implant therapy. As soon as we placed the temporary teeth, I could see that she was able to relax and felt comfortable smiling right away, she loved it. When she came back to get the permanent bridge, and saw how great it looked, how perfect and lovely her smile was, she was so happy that she started crying and thanking me.*

*She just loved the way it made her feel. She could smile with confidence and not have to worry about a denture moving or falling out when she ate. She could talk and laugh with her friends without being self-conscious. I'd say that if you rated her overall personal happiness in life before and after getting the bridge, on a scale from one to ten, she went from maybe three or to a nine. It was just a great result.*

## DENTAL BRIDGES

A dental bridge is a restorative process that dentists use to replace a missing tooth, multiple missing teeth or teeth that need to be extracted due to infection or breakage. The bridge consists of an artificial tooth or teeth that are permanently attached to the two adjacent teeth, which receive crowns, thus making a bridge. Bridges are three to five-part attachments: one or two or three artificial teeth that replace the missing ones, attached by crowns to two adjoining crowned teeth, one in front of the missing tooth/teeth and one behind. The bridge is cemented in like a traditional crown, which is then a permanent fixture within your mouth.

A bridge can be made of various materials, including metal, porcelain, or recently developed materials, such as zirconia (the same material as cubic zirconia that is used to create diamonds). The bridge is constructed to look, function, and feel just like natural teeth. Basically, the insertion of a bridge makes things exactly like they were before the tooth or teeth were lost, by restoring the function as well as a flawless smile.

A dental bridge is important for a person's function and health because it works to avoid some of the potential consequences of having a missing tooth, such as teeth shifting or food getting stuck in between the teeth where a tooth is missing. Plus, when you're missing a tooth, it can be uncomfortable or difficult for you to smile and eat and do all the normal things that you do. That's the main reason why it is very important to replace a missing tooth.

A dental bridge can also restore proper bite alignment, which is important in maintaining the health of the rest of your teeth since a poor bite can lead to tooth breakage or other problems such as gum disease.

## GETTING AND MAINTAINING A BRIDGE

The process of getting a bridge usually just takes a couple of visits. During the first visit, the dentist prepares the two teeth on either side of the missing tooth. The preparation involves removing a portion of enamel from those teeth for crowns to be placed over them (see the chapter on crowns). The dentist then takes an impression of the teeth, creating a model for a dental lab to use to make the bridge. The dentist also makes a temporary bridge for the patient to wear while the bridge is being created by the lab, which protects the exposed teeth and gums, and of course, also enables the patient to chew naturally and look whole again.

After the bridge is made by a dental lab, the patient returns for the dentist to remove the temporary one and replace it with the permanent bridge. The bridge fits exactly like a traditional single crown, except for the fact that the dentist is attaching three or more teeth together. Not often, but sometimes there may be a couple of follow-up visits needed for the dentist to check the bridge and adjust it to get the fit or the bite just right.

One thing that can lengthen the process a bit is if the patient needs bone grafting in the area of the missing tooth. If a tooth is extracted and a large defect is seen, bone graft should be placed to preserve the bone height and width. If a tooth has been missing for some time before the patient seeks to have it replaced with a bridge there may have been bone loss and bone grafting is necessary. Bone grafted to the defect left from the missing tooth, takes sometimes up to 6 months to heal properly. While you are waiting for the area to heal, the temporary bridge will serve to keep things stable. For either scenario, bone grafting repairs the bone structure of the jaw so that the bridge will fit solidly against the gums and is well-supported.

If a patient is missing more than one tooth, the process is still essentially the same for making a longer bridge. It just may require a couple of more visits and time, especially for any necessary extractions and bone grafting, to let the area heal, which will allow the proper fit of the bridge. It can take up to four appointments for a longer span bridge.

The longest bridge that a dentist will usually do is one that replaces three concurrently missing teeth, which means that five total teeth are involved when you include the two teeth on either end of the bridge that will serve as the anchor for the bridge. It's been my experience that trying to use a bridge for more than three missing teeth in a row results in a high incidence of fractures or breakage of the teeth involved. Even using a metal substructure, which is the strongest that we have, you get some flexure, so the bridge can move a bit under certain conditions. In any event, there's just a historically high failure rate with trying to bridge more than three missing teeth.

Once a patient has gotten a bridge, it's very important to keep the remaining teeth healthy and strong because the success of the bridge depends on a solid foundation being offered by the surrounding teeth. I'm careful to instruct my bridge patients on the importance of brushing, flossing, and using a fluoridated, or medicated, mouthwash daily to prevent tooth decay or gum (periodontal) disease. I also give patients cleaning tools, called proxy brushes, that are like little bottle brushes, which they can use to clean out food particles that may get underneath the bridge, or teeth.

A good dental bridge can last up to 25 years. How long a bridge lasts depends a lot on the patient's habits, such as whether they do things like chewing ice or grinding their teeth, as patients who grind their teeth typically break bridges more often. Depending on when a patient gets a bridge, it may last them the rest of their life, but in any event, the typical time is somewhere between five and 25 years, or about 15 years on average.

## ADVANTAGES AND DISADVANTAGES OF DENTAL BRIDGES

There are important advantages to replacing a missing tooth or teeth with a bridge. It enables you to chew and eat naturally, restores a proper bite alignment, and it's also esthetically appealing because it enables you to smile naturally and not be self-conscious about the appearance of your smile. Plus, you avoid the potential problems I mentioned about missing teeth, such as allowing other teeth to shift.

One advantage that a bridge offers over an alternative treatment such as getting a dental implant is that a bridge can be placed much more quickly, usually within a couple of weeks from start to finish. In contrast, a dental implant might take several months to do, and possibly involve going to both a specialist as well as a general dentist instead of just to the general dentist.

On the other hand, a disadvantage of a bridge, as compared to an implant, is that a bridge is harder to keep clean because of the fact that three or more teeth are bound together. Another potential disadvantage is that if one of the two teeth anchoring the bridge develops a cavity, the dentist may end up having to replace all three crowns (or four or five, depending on the length of the bridge) just because of that one cavity. Lastly, the bone and gum tissue under the missing tooth will, over time, recede or shrink, leaving a gap or space under the bridge. This can often lead to food impaction, discomfort and if in the front, unpleasing spaces.

There is one other disadvantage to using a bridge, and that's just the basic fact that you're treating one problem tooth but damaging two other healthy, virgin teeth. Those two teeth may be perfectly fine, but in order to do the bridge, you have to remove tooth structure and crown them just to hold the bridge in place.

## COST OF A BRIDGE

Most insurance plans cover a bridge restoration the same way they cover the cost of crowns. One possible financial obstacle for patients can be an annual insurance limit. For example, the maximum amount your dental insurance may offer to pay out in one year may equal about the cost of a single crown, but the cost of a bridge is usually the cost of three or more crowns, since that's essentially what the dentist is doing, crowning teeth.

Of course, there are several factors that can figure into the final cost, such as the cost of the lab that the dentist uses to manufacture the bridge as well as the type of material that will be used to fabricate the bridge. Most dentists offer a various types of finance plans to help their patients with any expenses not covered by a dental insurance plan.

## COSMETIC AND FUNCTIONAL BENEFITS FROM GETTING A BRIDGE

A bridge can be very esthetically pleasing. We can actually create bridges that look so natural you would never know that the patient ever had any teeth missing. People often forget that they have missing teeth, really.

Bridges can do so many wonderful things for patients. They can restore your smile, allow you to eat and speak properly, help to maintain an attractive shape to your face and jaw line, ensure a good bite alignment, and prevent more major dental problems that can develop from having missing teeth. A bridge can simply improve your life, through giving you a more beautiful smile. People who smile easily and often are happier, they tend to feel more awake and alert during the day, they're more self-confident, and they just generally feel better about themselves.

## DENTURES

A denture is a tooth replacement device made of acrylic, plasticized nylon, plastic, or metal that is fused to a mixture of these materials, which serves both functionally and in terms of restoring an appealing smile. There are also newer materials such as zirconia which are used to make permanent, implant supported, dentures. These newer materials are generally stronger and therefore longer lasting.

There are two types of dentures – complete and partial. A complete denture, which is what most people probably think of as dentures, is made of a removable plate that is used to replace every single tooth in a person's mouth. Partial dentures are just that – partial plates used to replace a number of missing teeth. They attach to the existing natural teeth, filling in the gaps left from missing teeth, and will function as normal teeth.

The primary reason for getting dentures is to replace teeth so that you can chew, eat, speak, and smile normally, but they also serve the purpose of reducing bone loss in the jaw that can occur when missing teeth are not replaced. Therefore, dentures also serve to maintain a healthy, attractive appearance. Dentists also make temporary dentures, full or partial, that are made to allow for healing after extractions or implant placement.

I show my patients a model that makes it easy for them to understand how important it is to maintain the bone structure of their mouth and jaw. The bones in the mouth are naturally shaped like a large "U". When teeth are missing and are not replaced by a denture or some other form of tooth replacement, that "U" shape, over time, narrows and becomes more like a "V" because the bones in our jaws gradually erode and shrink, both from side to side and from top to bottom.

That not only changes the shape and appearance of your face, but it also creates problems with actually being able to design a strong, solid tooth replacement with proper bite alignment and function for eating or talking, which makes placing implants, bridges or even dentures very difficult to use or place in your mouth. Dentures, or any other tooth replacement help to reduce bone loss and to support bite alignment, jaw and facial shape, and functionality for eating and talking.

## PARTIAL DENTURES AND WHOLE DENTURES

If you think back in time to your grandparents or someone else you knew with a partial denture, you may remember that when they smiled you could often see the metal retainers, or hooks, that attached to existing teeth. These days we can use acrylic materials to make the retainers, instead of metal, which gives a more esthetically desirable look. The retainers that do attach to existing teeth stabilize the denture to keep it from moving or falling out.

When the natural teeth are replaced with a whole denture, it's the gums and the underlying bones that are the support structure. For example, if you're missing all your teeth on top, the upper arch, a dental lab makes the denture in such a way that it gets suction, almost like a suction cup in the shower. You put the denture in and it holds on to your gums with suction and we can get a very good fit that way.

The bottom is somewhat different because you have to deal with both the tongue and the cheeks which are constantly moving and pushing on the denture. That makes it more difficult to maintain enough suction on the bottom to adequately hold the denture in place.

When my patients have a lot of problems with a lower arch, or bottom denture staying in place, I always discuss that it's better for the lower denture to have something to hold on to, such as existing teeth or implants, which will be the supporting structure for the denture.

## THE PROCESS OF GETTING DENTURES

The process of getting dentures usually entails about four or five visits to the dentist. Typically, patients, especially those getting whole dentures, need to have some teeth removed. Even patients getting a partial denture may need some decayed or loose teeth removed. For that reason, there's usually one visit before coming in for any necessary extractions

With multiple extractions, at that first visit, the dentist will take an impression and send that to a dental lab to create a temporary, or immediate denture for the patient to wear directly after the extractions, which are taken at a second visit approximately a week later. That temporary denture, which goes in right after any necessary extractions, acts as a pressure dressing while the patient's gums heal from the extractions. It covers the gums and holds pressure on them to allow the underlying bone to heal, allowing for much less shrinkage or recession of the supporting bone.

After the patient's mouth has healed – usually three to four months, although the healing time can vary from one patient to another – they come back, and it's during this third visit that the dentist takes a new impression and creates what we call a wax rim. That's essentially a dental substructure with wax on top of it. It's important for the dentist to check the dimensions, or distance of your jaws, between your nose and your chin.

This allows the dentist to make sure the denture won't put your jaws either too close together or too far apart, because either one of those conditions can interfere with your ability to speak naturally or chew food, as well as cause debilitating jaw joint, or TMJ, issues.

The next appointment involves putting in the wax rim, now with the artificial teeth set in it, and the dentist checking several other important things, such as how well the denture teeth occlude, or touch the other teeth in the mouth, which can be either with existing teeth or with another denture. We look at the bite alignment as well as the esthetics, or how nice the teeth look. Dentists do care about how the teeth are shaped and how the color matches either your existing teeth or your complexion. These are the same sort of checks a dentist makes when a patient gets a tooth crowned.

The next appointment is when the final denture is fit. After the wax rim is made and had the teeth set in it, then the dental lab uses that to create the final denture with a plasticized acrylic and the same teeth as far as color, shape, and size that were placed onto the wax rim.

After putting the final denture in, the dentist will check that there is good retention, or suction, for the denture, looking to see that it goes all the way down solidly onto the gums. In the case of a partial denture, we also want to check how solidly it attaches to existing teeth. We also check for places where the denture may push too hard so that it would cause pain or pressure sores.

When I adjust the denture, I usually tell my patients that the denture should feel almost like a gentle handshake – you should feel some pressure, but not discomfort and definitely not pain.

Virtually all patients need for the dentist to make some adjustments to the final denture to avoid sore spots, and that may require another few visits until they get the denture fit just right. There might be some pressure points that the patient doesn't notice right away when the denture first goes in, but that they notice within a week or two. When that happens I just have the patient come in and I make the necessary adjustments.

You clean a denture by taking it out of your mouth, rinsing off any food particles, and brushing it with your toothbrush. I generally recommend not to use toothpaste, because toothpaste has a fine grit, or a sandpaper effect that can cause scratches in the denture, which can cause it to discolor or more likely to hold food particles. I usually suggest that patients use either dish soap or hand soap with their toothbrush, and then, of course, rinse it thoroughly.

When patients remove dentures to let them soak for a thorough cleaning, they can use either an over-the-counter denture cleaning solution or a homemade one such as a mix of mouthwash, a little peroxide, and mostly water.

## ADVANTAGES AND DISADVANTAGES OF DENTURES

As dentists, we need to give all patients the various treatment options. A dentist is a healthcare provider, and while the patient should be in charge of their own healthcare, the more information that you have in terms of the various advantages and disadvantages, such as those provided in this book, the better choices you'll be able to make for treatment options.

If you're missing a single tooth, the first option would be a dental implant, a surgical component that interfaces with the bone of the jaw to support a crown (see the exciting chapter on implants). A second option is a bridge, where a dentist creates artificial teeth that attach to natural, existing, teeth adjacent to the missing tooth or teeth. A bridge can be used to replace up to three missing teeth in a row.

The third option, dentures, is what we go to when there are many missing teeth or teeth that need to be extracted, when a bridge isn't a workable option, when the patient either doesn't want or possibly can't afford dental implants, or as a healing option when multiple teeth are being replaced with implants, which would support the denture later on.

The advantages of getting dentures are that you can eat, you can smile, and can function normally. You are not losing the ability to eat your favorite foods, the ability to smile or to speak naturally. The process that we go through to make dentures, allows us to make them as natural as what God gave you, the only difference being that they're a removable prosthetic.

There are two primary disadvantages with dentures. One is that with a partial denture you can often see the hooks, metal or acrylic, that attach the denture to the existing teeth, and so that's not ideal for cosmetic purposes. The main problem with whole dentures is that they move over time, or become loose due to recession or bone shrinkage, and therefore need to be periodically replaced.

Dentures put pressure on the bone to help ease bone loss but it's not the same pressure that you get with chewing on natural teeth, so over time you still do experience some bone loss. That's why every five to ten years you usually have to get a new denture made in order for it to fit properly as the bone structure of your mouth changes.

It's different for each individual patient, because bone loss occurs at different rates and to different degrees in various people. I've seen people that need a new denture every couple of years, and then I've also seen people who haven't needed a new denture for 20 years.

Dentures can move or break, and they can also get lost since patients regularly take them out for cleaning. You don't have that problem with implants or bridges.

## DENTURE COSTS

One other advantage of dentures is affordability, particularly as compared to implants. We need to look at that as well as the health of the patient. If someone is not brushing their teeth regularly, not taking care good care of their teeth, a denture is a good option because you can take it out and clean it.

Most dental insurance covers dentures in the same way they cover bridges or crowns. Some insurance plans will pay for a new denture every five years; other plans may only pay for a new denture every eight years.

A complete set of whole dentures, upper and lower arch, ranges in cost from approximately $300 up to $5,000 per arch, in total $600 to $10,000. There's a pretty wide pricing range because there are several factors that can figure into the pricing, such as how much related work needs to done – things like how many extractions are needed or if implants are involved – and also because there's a wide range of quality.

The cheapest dentures are sort of "standard issue", premanufactured pieces that may not have the most cosmetically appealing look, these are usually the temporary or immediate dentures. Slightly more expensive dentures are custom-made, but usually with lower quality materials and lower quality warranties. Cheaper dentures are more prone to breakage and are usually thicker and heavier than the more expensive types, so they're less comfortable and less reliable.

Good quality, custom-made dentures typically cost in the neighborhood of $800 to $5,000 per arch. The most expensive dentures are those that are custom-made with the highest quality materials, which are lighter, less brittle and usually much stronger. These dentures usually come with excellent warranties that often include maintenance service. These are also the kind of dentures that are going to offer the best cosmetic look and are custom-made to give you your ideal smile.

For partial dentures, prices usually range from around $300 to $4,000 per denture, for the same reasons as seen above.

## DENTURES AND IMPLANTS

Sometimes dentists do a combination of implants and dentures. The implants provide a better support structure for dentures since they provide an anchor for the dentures to keep them from moving. If a patient has had multiple missing teeth for a long time, resulting in substantial bone loss, that makes a denture less stable, more prone to moving and to having something happen like the denture falling out when you open your mouth to talk or to laugh. An implant functions as a support anchor for the dentures, which solves that problem.

Implant supported dentures also offer the advantage of not having to rely on suction between the dentures and gums, allowing for a more natural feeling occlusion, or bite. Implant dentures are specially made to attach to the implants, some snapping into place and some screwed permanently into place.

Implant supported dentures are, however, more expensive. Prices can range from $3,000 up to $30,000 per arch.

## PATIENT SATISFACTION

A lot of patients I see, who are good candidates for dentures, are apprehensive. They may have seen older kinds of dentures that their grandparents had and they're worried about the look or about comfort or even the stigma that comes with wearing dentures. That's the time for me to help them get over any anxiety by talking with them and showing them how much the quality of dentures has improved over the years.

*I had one gentleman as a patient, a man in his late 50's. He was a salesman who was on the road all the time, talking to people and doing public speaking. He hadn't really taken care of his teeth to an ideal extent and as a result, he'd developed significant periodontal disease.*

*When I educated him that his best option was going to mean losing all of his teeth and getting complete dentures, he was devastated, but I walked him through it and was able to give him some reassurances. Fortunately, I had another denture patient in the office right then, so he was able to talk with her about her dentures and hear how happy she is with them.*

*With the dental technology that we have today, we can make dentures that look just like natural teeth and gums. So we went through the process of making a temporary denture, extracting his teeth, and eventually fitting him with the final, permanent denture, which was very natural-looking.*

*The day finally came that we gave him his final complete dentures and he was hesitant. But he ended up being really ecstatic about how good they looked, and he came back a couple of days later just to tell me, "Thank you - because I can talk, I can eat, I can smile. I don't have to worry about my teeth falling out anymore. I was so worried about losing my job because most of my work is done by talking to people and taking them out for lunch."*

That's usually the way things go with patients. They're apprehensive or scared at first, but when they finally get the dentures, the dentures look great! They have the best-looking smile they've had in years, and their ability to eat and speak naturally is restored, they're usually just very, very grateful for what we're able to do for them with a good quality denture.

# ABOUT JACOB DEVINNEY, DDS

Amador Dental & Orthodontic
AmadorDental.com

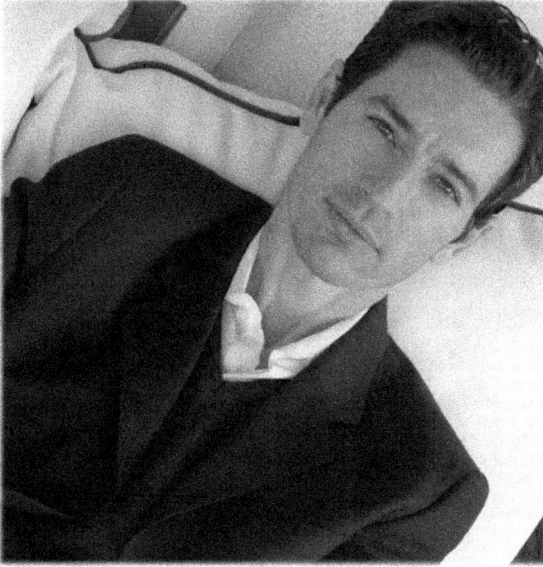

Dr. Jacob DeVinney is a caring and talented professional who is committed to providing the highest quality dental care to his patients. He brings years of experience to his Pleasanton practice, and as the new owner of Amador Dental and Orthodontic, is committed to offering safe and comfortable dental procedures to his patients and to providing continuity of care throughout the Pleasanton area. He continues Amador Dental and Orthodontic's tradition of creating a positive and compassionate climate where patients feel welcome and in offering the latest in cutting-edge dental technology for the best results possible.

Dr. "Jake" DeVinney served six years in the United States Navy as an ENT surgical technician and Hospital Corpsman before attending Cal State University, Dominguez Hills, where he earned a BS in Biology. He then went on to attend USC's Herman Ostrow School of Dentistry, where he attained his DDS.

Dr.   DeVinney    keeps up-to-date through    endless training, including professional development, which is designed to teach the latest breakthroughs and advances in dental technology.

Above all, Dr. DeVinney is committed to creating a great patient experience. He offers thorough explanations to his patients of any necessary dental procedures and answers all dental health questions with honesty and integrity. As a provider of both adult and pediatric dental services, he offers exceptional dental care for the entire family. He relies on a team of caring and committed professionals to provide a comfortable and supportive atmosphere where the patient's needs always come first. As a premier Pleasanton dentist, Dr. DeVinney brings enthusiasm and expertise to better serve his patients and his community.

# REPLACING YOUR TEETH WITH DENTAL IMPLANTS

Going to the dentist is not a favorite activity for most of my patients. Having a surgical procedure is certainly even less desired. So to say to patients that dental implants are one of the most exciting dental advances of all time is not always met with enthusiasm - unless, of course, you are suffering from one or more missing teeth!

Loss of a tooth, multiple teeth or even all teeth can have many undesirable consequences, such as the following:

- Embarrassment
- Loss of confidence
- Less smiling and laughing
- Loss of chewing of favorite foods
- Premature aging face
- Loss of work or career
- Less intimacy

Losing a tooth or teeth often leads to a decrease in the quality of life. As an Oral & Maxillofacial surgeon, it is such a pleasure and honor to give my patients back the quality of life they want and deserve. Dental implants are today's best and most advanced man-made solution for replacing teeth. In fact, there are very few replacement "body parts" today that look, function and feel so much like the original.

The good news is that a missing tooth is not a heart valve. Unlike a heart, you can survive without a tooth or teeth. But if you are experiencing any of the consequences listed above, you don't have to suffer like your grandparents may have.

The best part of being an implant surgeon is the feedback I get once treatment is complete. Here are some of the comments that I've gotten from implant patients:

- "That was so much easier than I expected!"
- "I love my new smile!"
- "I can eat whatever I want"
- "I wish I had done this sooner!"
- "It has changed my life!"

Here's just one story of the awesome difference that getting dental implants made in the life of one of my patients:

*Betty was a 55-year-old mother of three whose life was once turned upside down because of her failing teeth. When I first met Betty, she talked very little and avoided eye contact, looking mostly at the floor. She constantly pulled her hair forward to cover her mouth. Her general physical appearance reflected that she had all but given up on the way she looked, a fact that she confirmed.*

*The look of her teeth had even begun to drastically affect her familial relationships – she told me that she no longer remained in contact with her children. It was obvious that she suffered from extremely low self-esteem, depression, and had serious anxiety issues when in public settings. After the first examination, I understood why. Betty's teeth were severely damaged and decayed. She had consistently noticeably bad breath and was in constant pain.*

*After replacing her upper and lower teeth with the ReVita Smile® implant treatment (All-on-Four®, immediate full arch dental implant treatment), Betty's life was completely transformed. She loves her life again and her outlook and perspective have changed tremendously. Her whole personality is different now. She's confident, enjoys social interactions, and has rebuilt her relationships with family members. She started taking care of herself again, changing her hair, wearing makeup, and revamping her wardrobe as well. She smiles constantly and makes eye contact when speaking with others.*

Of all the patients I've seen, Betty's story is one that has touched everyone at my office. The drastic effect that a one-day treatment had on this woman was more than any of us expected - it completely transformed her life. My office staff and I couldn't be happier with Betty's results. It makes me feel proud, but more than that, it's the reason that I do what I do.

Everyone enjoys an improved quality of life and is happy to get their teeth back. I would like to share and emphasize the important fact: not all dental implants surgeons, restorative doctors, dental implant companies, dental labs, dental implant techniques and even patients are created equal. There are variables that can and do affect treatment and the end result. An important part of my practice is to educate patients and aid patients in obtaining the best possible outcome.

## THE BASICS OF DENTAL IMPLANTS

It's important for patients to understand what dental implants are. Dental implants are man-made tooth root replacements. Typically, dental implants are made with mostly titanium, which is a popular bio-compatible metal used for reconstruction of body parts, such as hip replacements.

The dental implant is placed into the jawbone and heals through a process called "osseointegration", usually within 2 to 5 months ("Osseo" refers to bone and "integration" refers to accepting the implant as part of the bone.) During this time, the bone heals much like a broken bone heals and the implant becomes secured in the bone such that it is strong enough to support a single tooth crown, multiple teeth (a bridge), or even a full set of teeth. The most popular dental implant design is a screw-type. The beauty of dental implants is that they look and function as a natural tooth.

## THE HISTORY OF IMPLANTS

The dental implant, like so many other great discoveries, was completely accidental. In the early 1960's, a physician named Dr. Per Ingar Branemark was completing a study to evaluate bone healing. Dr. Branemark implanted hollow titanium screws into rabbit leg bones with a viewing window. He observed bone healing at different phases through this window and recorded his findings. Upon completion of the study, Dr. Branemark went to remove the titanium screws but was fascinated to learn that they were fused to the bone and could not be easily removed.

The doctor spent many of the next years studying this phenomenon. Initially, he intended to study the use of titanium replacements for hips and other parts of the body but transitioned his studies to the mouth because it was easier to observe clinically. Branemark published a number of studies based on his observations and eventually commercialized a dental implant system in 1981.

Today, with advanced technology, the process of developing realistic-looking teeth using dental implants continues to grow and change. Characteristically, earlier teeth restored using dental implants were bulkier and more artificial looking due to limited materials and knowledge with regard to shaping and attaching artificial teeth to the tops of the implanted screws. Doctors are now able to match the shape and color to a patient's original teeth to give them a much more realistic look, or to custom-design brand new, bright white teeth to give their patients a perfect and beautiful smile.

## THE NEED FOR DENTAL IMPLANTS

There are a variety of situations that warrant the need for dental implants or situations where I would recommend them for my patients. Simply put, anyone missing one, multiple, or all teeth should consider dental implants. This is not to say that every tooth needs to be replaced with an implant. However, when replacement of a tooth is desired, dental implants have significant benefits over traditional dental options. There are a number of factors to consider in regard to getting implants.

## FACTORS TO CONSIDER – OVERALL MEDICAL HEALTH

Generally speaking, patients considering dental implants should be in good overall health and have any ongoing medical conditions well-managed. Poor health and unhealthy lifestyles can lead to unfavorable outcomes with any surgical or dental procedure and dental implants are no exception to this fact.

Dental implants are not "superheroes" that can survive in any type of health and, like teeth, they can fail due to poor health. Patients with common medical conditions such as diabetes, heart conditions, osteoporosis, or autoimmune diseases, once controlled and well managed by a physician, can enjoy the benefits of dental implants. Smoking is a special consideration, as it is harmful to both your general and dental health. Many patients who smoke have successful dental implants but the treatment is typically more challenging.

Two special medical situations require more attention are patients that receive radiation treatment to the jaws ( i.e. for cancer treatment) or patients taking medication for osteoporosis. Either of these situations may interfere with bone healing and therefore need special consideration before getting dental implants.

## FACTORS TO CONSIDER - DENTAL HEALTH

While dental implants are not at risk of getting decayed or ever needing a root canal, they do need healthy bone and gum tissue for long-term success. It is important to obtain and maintain a mouth without gum disease and decayed teeth, as well as to have a good, well-aligned "bite." Sometimes it is necessary to treat and manage other dental problems before replacing missing teeth with dental implants. Routine and regular hygiene, as well as professional dental care, is required with dental implants just as with natural teeth.

## FACTORS TO CONSIDER - ANATOMY

Dental implants rely on the existing jawbone and tissue for support and health. Loss of teeth is generally associated with the loss or shrinkage of the jawbone. Additionally, everyone also has their own unique anatomy of the jaws, which can vary in size, shape, and density. The upper jaw has the maxillary sinuses above the back teeth and the lower jaw has nerves which need to be avoided to prevent nerve damage.

Fortunately, today's advanced technology enables us to do an excellent job of evaluating a patient's jaw anatomy and, thereby, enhancing the chances for success. For patients with inadequate bone or tissue, grafting is available to enhance the anatomy and to allow for placement of dental implants.

## FACTORS TO CONSIDER - FINANCIAL

Generally, dental implants are not the least expensive option for replacing missing teeth. However, dental implants do usually provide a superior quality of life as patients receiving implants can avoid concerns about teeth moving or falling out, collecting food while eating, or being conscientious when you speak, eat, smile or laugh.

Dental implants are an investment in your quality of life, your confidence, health, and enjoyment. Still, your dental budget is important, just as with purchasing a car, and should be addressed when considering dental implants. At this time, implants are not typically covered by insurance plans, but dentists are aware of this, so many of them offer financing plans for patients.

## POSSIBLE CONSEQUENCES OF NOT GETTING IMPLANTS

There are a variety of negative consequences of missing teeth for patients choosing not to get dental implants. One such consequence is bone and tissue shrinkage, otherwise known as atrophy. Once the tooth has been extracted, a "socket" results in the jawbone where the tooth roots existed. The socket becomes filled with a blood clot and wound healing immediately begins. The bone socket heals like a broken bone. The blood clot creates a matrix for bone cells from the blood to collect and begin bone healing. The bone around the socket is no longer supported by the tooth root and begins to contract or shrink to eliminate the bone defect. Initially, there is significant bone shrinkage and then a defect results. Unfortunately, shrinkage of the bone and tissue continues to occur over time, much like a slowly melting ice cube. This process of bone "melting away" is called atrophy.

Other possible treatments, such as bridges or dentures, accelerate loss of teeth and bone, which can eventually make it difficult, if not impossible, for a patient to receive dental implants. To place a bridge, the natural teeth next to missing teeth must be cut down to place crowns. The natural teeth offer support for the replacement artificial teeth and take on more of the chewing forces.

There are potential problems with bridges. It is difficult to clean under a bridge, which may cause decay to develop on one or more of the supporting teeth. The additional forces and recurrent decay may lead to an earlier loss of the supporting teeth and may trigger the vicious cycle of tooth loss and bone shrinkage.

Partial dentures are removable replacement teeth that hook to existing teeth for support with clasps. A problem with this treatment is that, besides being aesthetically undesirable, the clasps may lead to loss of the anchor teeth over time. A complete denture replaces a full arch of missing teeth and sits directly on the gum tissue. The bone and tissue under a partial or complete denture usually suffer from accelerated bone shrinkage due to the continual chewing forces the dentures place on the jaws.

## PLACEMENT OF DENTAL IMPLANTS

In some cases, a tooth can be removed and the dental implant placed at the same time, or a tooth might already be missing and an implant ready for immediate placement. In those scenarios, there is typically one procedure with two follow-up visits, and then one or two more visits to make and deliver the crown, bridge or final teeth. In other situations, the tooth needs to be removed and time allowed for the site to heal – usually 2 to 6 months – and then the implant may be placed.

If a tooth is already missing but inadequate bone is present, bone grafting might be completed and the implant placed after the graft heals, typically in 3 to 5 months. In those scenarios, two procedures are completed with follow-up appointments, followed by delivery of the crown, bridge or final teeth.

In cases where a full arch of teeth needs removal or is missing, the dental implants and a full arch of non-removable temporary teeth may all be placed in one procedure, in just one day. There will be a couple of preliminary visits to prepare and some follow-up appointments to make the final bridge.

It is important to realize that, like any medical or surgical procedure, not everything works 100% of the time. Fortunately, research and data have shown that the success rate of dental implants is 94% to 96% in the upper jaw and 96% to 98% in the lower jaw. There are very few medical and dental procedures that enjoy such high success rates.

Total implant treatment times are usually 3 to 6 months from start to finish. In some cases, treatment may be as little as 10 weeks, and in other cases, it may take up to one year. When desired, especially in the front teeth, a temporary tooth may be provided while the dental implant is healing.

## MAINTENANCE OF DENTAL IMPLANTS

Dental implants will never develop decay or need a root canal, but they do need healthy teeth and gums for long-term success. With good medical and dental health, dental implants may last a lifetime. Of all dental techniques and procedures offered in dentistry, dental implants generally have the most favorable prognosis. With some restorations, there may be noticeable wear and tear or staining over time. It is possible that the restoration on the implants – the crown or bridge placed – may need repair or replacement at some time in the future.

Taking good care of dental implants is vital to making them last and is the same as caring for natural teeth. Brushing, flossing and irrigating with water is a must. It's important for patients to practice good dental hygiene and to see their dentist on an ongoing basis. Dentists use special instruments when cleaning implants to avoid damaging them.

## FINDING THE RIGHT SURGEON FOR DENTAL IMPLANTS

It's important for patients to ask questions before choosing a surgeon to do implants. Find out what type of implant system they use – there are hundreds available – and get statistics on how successful that particular implant system has been. The most important thing to know is the skill level of the surgeon. Find out how and where the surgeon got his or her education. Some surgeons have had years of intensive training in graduate programs while others have only attended "weekend" training programs. Ask your implant surgeon how long they've been surgically placing dental implants and how often they perform implant surgery.

*One patient I treated, Mark, played in a softball league. He was playing with his team days before his wedding. During the game he was hit in the face by the ball, fracturing his two front teeth down to the gum line. He contacted my office for emergency care and in a panic as his wedding was in a few days!*

*Working closely with his restorative dentist, we developed a plan to have him ready for his wedding. After sedating him, I removed the fractured, non-repairable teeth and immediately placed two dental implants with bone grafting. During the same appointment, I placed custom posts to allow the restorative doctor to provide replacement crowns that blended seamlessly into his natural smile on the same day.*

*Using advanced digital dental technology and working closely with the patient's own dentist, he was awake, alert, with beautiful, non-removable new front teeth within a few hours. He attended his wedding with a gorgeous smile, pain-free and no one was the wiser. Now this story had a happy ending partially because Mark chose the right dental surgeon and implant team as many would not be able to offer the same treatment.*

## EDUCATION AND COLLABORATION

It's vital that an implant surgeon remains a perpetual student because little to none of the knowledge needed to do implants is taught in dental school. I suggest that anyone considering implants should find a surgeon that has gotten at least three or more years of additional surgical training after they've finished dental school.

As an Oral & Maxillofacial surgeon, I spent years studying surgical techniques that ranged from simple tooth removal to complete facial bone and tissue reconstruction before I entered into private practice. Years of surgical training provides extensive knowledge of anatomy, managing complications, and anesthesia techniques.

Getting implants is a two-step process that requires collaboration and teamwork between a surgeon and a restorative dentist. Education is key and plays a large part of why I offer continuing education to dentists on a host of implant and surgery aspects. This allows the collaboration process to flow more seamlessly.

Once an oral surgeon has placed the implants, the patient then follows up with a general or restorative dentist who possesses expertise in fillings, crowns, veneers, bridges, dentures – the aesthetic part of the implant.

This is not to say that general or restorative dentists can't and don't sometimes take care of the entire implant process. However, most dentists don't perform implant surgery often and if they do, it is usually the most difficult and complex service they offer. In my experience, it's best to complete the process with a surgical specialist and a restorative dentist that value collaboration and working together to obtain the best possible results. This allows each doctor to perform where they excel in their respective fields and provide the most favorable outcome for the patient.

## NEW TECHNOLOGY AND TECHNIQUES

The field of dental implants is constantly changing and developing. Digital technology is quickly improving the predictability and outcome of dental implants. One of the most important developments in recent years is the 3D x-ray, also called a Cone-Beam Computed Tomography (CBCT) scan. This enables an implant surgeon to view and identify bone volume, contour, and vital structures such as nerves and the sinuses. These x-rays provide critical information for a surgeon to map out and precisely plan implant placement, avoiding undesirable complications. The information offered by 3D x-rays allows a surgeon to make better surgical choices, which in turn lead to better short and long-term results for the patient.

Another advancement in the digital world involves merging of 3D x-rays and digitally generated impressions, where a camera is used to generate a digital impression instead of an impression using the "goop" which so many patients dislike. The information gathered enables a surgeon to recreate your entire mouth and head on the computer and perform "virtual surgery". This makes it possible for a surgeon to identify ideal results and complete "run-through" of the implant surgery before ever touching the patient. The surgeon can identify and note ideal positions and placement for implants, as well as mark trouble spots and areas to be avoided.

In my practice, we also utilize a 3-D printer to fabricate a surgical guide that allows for precise placement of dental implants as planned for in the "virtual surgery." Utilizing digital dental technology is advanced and most surgeons do not have the training or knowledge to offer such progressive treatment. My philosophy is to use advanced digital technology to obtain the best possible results for every implant, in every patient, no matter how simple or complex the case. I certainly would want the best results in my mouth every time!

Once the surgery is complete, digital technology can be used, again, to provide excellent results. When "testing" dental implants to confirm adequate and successful healing, a digital impression is taken during this follow up visit. A digital shade is also obtained to create the most accurate tooth color to match the existing teeth. This impression is sent to the restorative dentist to design and plan the custom implant supported teeth on the computer. This inevitably saves the patient time (less visits and less time at the office) and generally leads to the most aesthetically-pleasing smile.

## *ReVita* Smile® (All-on-Four® Treatment Concept)

*ReVita* Smile®, often referred to as the All-on-Four® treatment concept, is a newer and advanced treatment technique in which a full arch of unhealthy teeth is removed, dental implants placed and beautiful, non-removable teeth placed in just one procedure. *ReVita* Smile® also allows patients wearing dentures to have non-removable teeth in just one day.

Patients tend to have confusion how this procedure is possible. The primary concept making this possible is cross-arch stabilization. This means that when you bite or chew on this new bridge of teeth, the force is evenly distributed throughout the entire bridge so that none of the implants are overloaded. This is different from a shorter bridge, or single crown, where all the forces of your bite bear down directly on the newly placed implants.

This technique also makes it possible for more patients to receive dental implants. Oftentimes, a patient is told they don't have enough bone for an implant. In terms of traditional implants, maybe this is true, but it is rarely the case with *ReVita* Smile® treatment, which uses the best available bone to secure the final bridge, replacing both the crown of the tooth and the gums. Because both are replaced, dental implants can be inserted in various locations – the area of the jawbone with the thickest and most stable bone – to support a bridge without needing any bone grafting or multiple surgeries.

*ReVita* Smile® is truly one of the most fascinating and rewarding of implant treatments I provide. It is a pleasure to see patients end years of frustration with pain, dental failure and years of ongoing dental disease. Patients immediately begin to smile and speak, and ultimately eat, with confidence. In just one procedure on just one day, *ReVita* Smile® changes patients' lives!

## SUCCESS STORY OF DENTAL IMPLANTS - *REVITA* SMILE®

Getting dental implants can be a wonderful experience for patients, one that totally changes their life. Patients will often wait for a special time in their life before they will reach out for help. The moment they do a success story is born.

*Another groom-to-be patient I had was Jared. He was a hardworking 33-year-old who came to see me about two months before his engagement pictures were to be taken. He was incredibly self-conscious about his smile and told me that all he wanted was a new smile for this new stage of his life. He just wanted to look good and smile big at his bride when she walked down the aisle.*

*Though fairly young and in good health otherwise, Jared had a number of missing teeth, and those that remained had advanced decay. His long history as a smoker and lack of dental care was the primary culprit. He complained of constant pain and difficulty chewing as he had so much decay in teeth on his upper and lower jaws.*

*I was able to perform a ReVita Smile® reconstructive surgery to replace his teeth and eliminate the pain and difficulty chewing. He had the beautiful wedding he dreamed of and things went smoothly as planned. He couldn't be happier and smiles all the time now. He reported being able to explore new foods and new restaurants with his wife, something he wouldn't have been able to do without the ReVita Smile®. His quality of life has improved significantly. It is not an exaggeration to say that getting implants really turned his life around for the better.*

I strongly urge people who have missing teeth or other severe dental problems to talk with their dentist and explore the possibilities of dental implants. Implants are a major technological advance in dentistry and can provide patients with truly miraculous cosmetic results.

## ABOUT DR. SCOTT FRANK

North Shore Oral & Maxillofacial Surgery
SmileSurgery.com

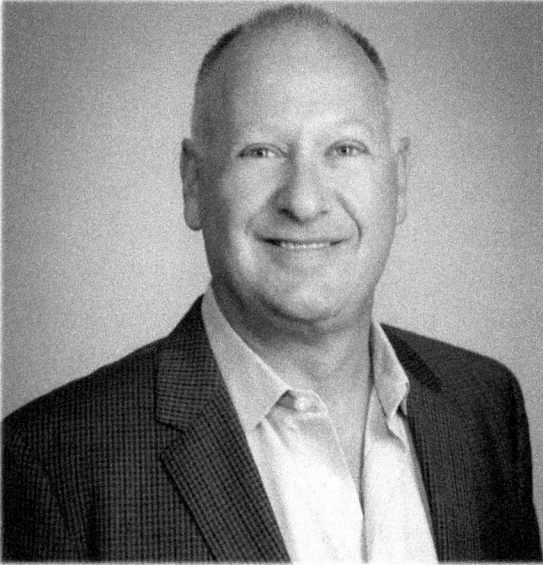

A Chicago native, Dr. Scott Frank has been bringing his talent and expertise to the "Chicagoland" for almost 30 years. During this time, he has earned elite status with numerous accolades while serving the needs of thousands of patients.

Born and raised in Chicago, Dr. Frank attended the University of Illinois, Champaign-Urbana, for his undergraduate studies in engineering. He received his Doctorate of Dental Surgery degree from Northwestern University in 1987 and was selected for an externship at the University of Chicago Hospital that focused on cancers of the head and neck. He also completed an extensive residency in Oral & Maxillofacial Surgery at Howard University Hospital in Washington, D.C.

While at Howard University Hospital, he received extensive facial and dentoalveolar surgical experience which focused on extraction, bone and tissue grafts, dental implant reconstruction, infections and trauma. This led to his lifelong interest in hard and soft tissue reconstructive surgery, sinus and regenerative bone grafts, the safe and effective removal of teeth, as well as smile enhancement utilizing dental implants.

Dr. Frank is passionate about continuing his education and attends more than 100 hours of classes courses sponsored by accredited organizations each year. He enjoys sharing his knowledge by educating his peers on dental implant restorative techniques, particularly Digital Implant Dentistry and *ReVita* Smile® procedures, of which he has currently performed nearly 1,000. He has also organizes many continuing education programs for local doctors, offering his expertise regularly as a speaker, mentor and leader. He has been accredited by the Academy of General Dentistry to award educational units for courses presented by North Shore Oral & Maxillofacial Surgery.

In addition to his work with continuing education, Dr. Frank has served since 2001 as the Director of the Elite Dental Group, a local chapter of the prestigious Seattle Study Club, an interactive group focused on interdisciplinary and comprehensive dentistry. He is also a member of the American Association of Oral & Maxillofacial Surgeons, the American Dental Association, the Illinois State Dental Society, the Chicago Dental Society and the Academy of Osseointegration, as well as a fellow of the International Congress of Oral Implantologist.

Dr. Frank has unusually extensive experience with *ReVita* Smile®, often referred to as the All-on-Four® treatment concept. In this procedure, a patient receives an entire set of upper and/or lower teeth in a single visit. He is also unique as he uses advanced digital dental technology to ensure the best possible outcome for all patients. As part of the North Shore Oral & Maxillofacial

Surgery, Dr. Frank and his team provide quality, professional dental surgery to ensure all his patients throughout the Chicago area and from throughout the US receive the most exceptional experience. Visit www.SmileSurgery.com for further information about Dr. Frank, his team and his practice.

SHITAL PATEL, DDS
AND RAKESH PATEL, DDS

# NO FEAR WITH SEDATION DENTISTRY

Sedation dentistry is a simple and safe technique used to enable many dental patients to receive necessary cosmetic, or other dental treatment they want by feeling more comfortable and relaxed. It can be especially helpful if you're a patient who may have high anxiety levels about having dental work done. Here's how sedation dentistry helped one person obtain that beautiful smile they'd always wanted:

A lady in her fifties, whom we'll call "Mary," came to us when she was very badly in need of some major dental work. She hadn't been to a dentist in a very long time, and her front teeth were all broken down, and she had several other problems too. She was so self-conscious about the way her teeth looked that she hardly ever smiled. She was the kind of person who, if she did smile or grin, would cover her mouth with her hand. And the main reason that she had put off getting dental work done was her anxiety about having all the necessary procedures.

What finally prompted her to come in was the fact that her sister had apparently gotten a lot of successful dental work done recently, and so that made Mary feel more confident that she could get her teeth properly fixed, too. She felt like it was the right time in her life to get things taken care of, but she still had some basic anxiety issues about the whole thing.

I met with her, and at the end of my examination I explained to her that she was in need of multiple root canals and crowns, as well as some extractions. She basically needed to get all her teeth crowned, because there was so much damage. To handle her anxiety issues, I explained to her about sedation dentistry and told her I felt that using sedation, where we could do a lot of work in one visit, was the best option.

Using intravenous sedation, we were able to take care of everything in just two visits. The first visit took about four hours and the second visit just a couple of hours, and in those two visits, we completely changed her smile. That was about six years ago, and she comes in now for regular hygiene visits, and she just looks beautiful. And now she smiles – beams – all the time, which is a wonderful thing to see. It's not saying too much to say that it's really changed her whole attitude in terms of how she sees herself and how others see her. She is more confident and more comfortable when she is interacting with people. She's really a completely different person. You can't put a price tag on something like that. So, that's what sedation dentistry can do for someone, and that's why I'm so thankful that we're able to offer it.

On a purely personal level, it's just wonderful for me as a dentist to be able to help patients make such a beautiful, awesome change in how a person feels about themselves. And that's why I wish more patients knew about sedation dentistry and how it can help them get that amazing smile that can really change their whole lives. One of the most remarkable things is how quickly we can make that happen for them. Think about it – all those years of neglect, and pain, and all that time spent self-consciously not smiling, and we were able to fix all of that, to just turn her life completely around, in just six hours of dental work. And thanks to sedation dentistry, even though she had some dental anxiety issues beforehand, she was completely comfortable all that time, no problems at all.

That's just one example of how the "magic" of sedation dentistry can help patients make a really positive change in their lives.

Why is sedation dentistry so important? – Basically because of the fact that a fairly large number of people suffer from dental phobia or anxiety. It's estimated that up to 15% - or about 30 to 40 million people in the U.S. – avoid getting needed dental work done because of dental anxiety. About one-third of people who don't visit a dentist regularly say that fear or anxiety is the main reason they avoid going to a dentist. So if you happen to suffer from dental anxiety, you're not alone.

Because dental fear causes people to avoid going to the dentist, that leads to higher risk of gum disease and tooth loss. And dental anxiety can cause other problems besides just dental problems. People who have damaged or discolored teeth, and who need some major cosmetic dentistry, are often very self-conscious, or embarrassed, about their smile. That puts stress on them by making them feel insecure, especially in social situations. A lot of people lack self-esteem because they lack a beautiful smile, and that can affect their lives both personally and professionally.

That's why sedation dentistry, which is specifically designed to help people deal with dental anxiety, can be so important and helpful to you if you're someone who would really like to take care of some major dental problems, but you've held back because of some anxiety about having dental work done. Sedation dentistry can be just the thing to help you finally take care of all your dental problems and get that perfect, beautiful smile you've always wanted.

## WHAT IS SEDATION DENTISTRY?

Sedation dentistry is basically just about using medication to help people with dental anxiety handle getting dental work done.

There are three basic techniques used to provide sedation dentistry. The first, and simplest, option uses the administration of nitrous oxide, commonly referred to as "laughing gas". Nitrous oxide sedation is often the most appropriate choice when a patient is just having a simple procedure done that takes relatively little time. It's very safe and controlled, and patients can usually drive themselves home on the same day with no problems. Nitrous oxide is a commonly used procedure for patients who experience high anxiety levels with even the most basic dental procedures, such as a cleaning.

Another option is oral sedation, where the patient takes either sedative liquids or tablets. Oral sedation is useful when a patient is having a sizeable amount of dental work done, such as a root canal, for example.

The third means of sedation is intravenous, or IV, sedation. This procedure is handled by an anesthesiologist who administers the sedation and also monitors the patient throughout the time their dental work is being done. A key advantage of IV sedation is that it allows for more dental work to be completed in a single visit. Many patients prefer getting a lot of work over and done with in just one visit to the dentist, rather than going in several times.

If you're having either IV or oral sedation, you'll need to arrange to have someone to drive you home after the visit, since it may take a few hours for the sedation to wear off completely, and therefore it's just not safe for you to be driving.

## THINGS TO CONSIDER WHEN YOU HAVE SEDATION DENTISTRY

There are some things you may want to consider in making a choice for sedation dentistry. One of the main things is how time-consuming or complex is the work you're having done. For relatively simple procedures that don't take much time to complete, you may want to go with the simplest and most basic sedation method, nitrous oxide. If you want to get some more involved work done, work that might take more than an hour to complete, then you may be more inclined to look at getting oral or IV sedation.

The cost might be a factor in your decision, too. Due to insurance limitations, or other reasons, you may decide that IV sedation is just cost-prohibitive for you. You might opt for nitrous oxide sedation because it's the least expensive method, the recovery time is shorter, and you probably won't need to bring a "chaperone" along to drive you home.

Also to consider is the fact that IV sedation simply may not be a practical option for you because of the fact that relatively few dental offices offer it. We do offer IV sedation as an option in our practice, but there are only about 10% of dental offices offering IV sedation. That's because the IV sedation requires having an anesthesiologist on hand to administer it and monitor the procedure. Oral sedation is more commonly available. It does require special training for the dentist, but it doesn't require the services of an anesthesiologist or all the extra monitoring equipment necessary for doing IV sedation.

We also sometimes do a combination of nitrous oxide and oral sedation. In some instances, we might start a patient off with nitrous oxide, and then if while we're doing the procedure, we determine that more sedation is optimal, then we can move to oral sedation. It also might happen the other way round, starting off with oral sedation and then adding some nitrous oxide just to provide a bit more effective level of sedation to make the patient more comfortable.

The most important factor in making a decision to use sedation dentistry, and what specific sedation procedure to employ, is your personal anxiety level. We want to make the dental procedure as easy and comfortable for each individual patient as possible. It's ultimately you, the patient, who makes the decision, and we just want to make sure that we do the best job we can of making you aware of the options, so that you can make a sound, informed decision that you feel is best for you.

In our experience, with patients who opt for some form of sedation dentistry, approximately 70-80% choose oral sedation, and probably another 15% prefer IV sedation. The nitrous oxide option is less commonly selected, but it may be the best choice, as noted earlier, for relatively simple procedures that can be completed in a short amount of time.

I should mention that nitrous oxide is an excellent option when working with children who may naturally have some level of anxiety. In my experience, a little bit of nitrous often just makes it significantly easier to perform dental work on kids.

## WHEN TO CONSIDER SEDATION DENTISTRY

Sedation dentistry is most commonly useful for helping patients who, for one reason or another, have a high level of dental anxiety. What we often find is that someone has had a past experience that causes them to have a high level of anxiety about getting dental work done, and that this has prevented them from having procedures done – they've just pretty much tried to avoid going to a dentist because of their anxiety. Also, if you haven't been going to the dentist regularly, and have a lot of dental work that needs to be done, work that will likely take a considerable amount of time to complete, that makes considering sedation dentistry even more appropriate.

And you may just prefer having everything done in a single visit. A lot of people do, just because they have very busy schedules or work or family commitments that make it difficult for them to arrange multiple appointments. If for example, you have a few cavities or some gum problems, then one visit with oral sedation may be ideal.

Wisdom teeth extractions and dental implants are procedures where sedation dentistry is highly appropriate, and we often find that IV sedation is the best option to go with in those cases, as long as the patient is comfortable with that choice. This is especially true in cases where you're having multiple implants done, which often involves bone grafting.

## MEDICAL CONSIDERATIONS

Before making a decision to use sedation dentistry, we always take into consideration any medical issues a patient may have. For example, patients who are pregnant can't ordinarily have any type of sedation. In fact, pregnancy is probably the number one factor that would make a patient not a good candidate for sedation dentistry. There are other medical conditions, such as high blood pressure, where we'd get clearance from your doctor before using any sedation, and obviously, we abide by whatever determination your healthcare provider makes. However, in the majority of cases, there's no medical problem with using any of the sedation dentistry techniques.

Since we always want to go with whatever you as an individual patient are most comfortable with, your preference is often the deciding factor. Some patients, for example, simply don't like needles at all, and so using IV sedation would, in fact, increase their anxiety level. Now, in some of those cases – situations where IV sedation appears to be advisable – what we can do is start off with oral sedation, and then once the patient is more relaxed, we can administer the IV sedation.

A lot of patients simply aren't aware that oral sedation even exists as an option, and once we explain it to them, many of them immediately respond with, "Yeah, that sounds great to me. Let's go with that."

## COST CONSIDERATIONS

Cost is typically a major consideration for many patients regarding sedation dentistry. If you're a patient who's in need of multiple extractions, root canals, or fillings, that might make you an ideal patient to consider having IV sedation. However, an anesthesiologist may charge up to $600-$700 an hour, so that can add significantly to the total cost of getting your dental work done. Nitrous oxide sedation generally only costs around $80 to $150 total, and oral sedation usually ranges from about $150 to $250.

Insurance coverage for sedation dentistry is, unfortunately, often unclear. With a lot of PPO plans, the plan only covers IV sedation if the procedure involves multiple extractions, implants, or similar work.

Actually, because of the maximum benefit allowances on most insurance plans, it's a moot point as far as whether the insurance will specifically cover the sedation. For example, if you're having four wisdom teeth removed, or a couple of root canals done, the cost of the dental work itself usually exceeds the insurance plan's maximum annual benefit, so there's no insurance coverage remaining to cover the cost of sedation anyway.

One thing that can sometimes help is seeing if your medical insurance coverage, rather than dental insurance, will cover at least part of the cost. We try to do the best job possible of defraying your out of pocket expenses or helping out with payment plans so that you don't have to cover all of the cost at one time.

## TIME CONSIDERATIONS

Since sedation dentistry is commonly used in conjunction with doing multiple dental procedures, it typically applies to dental visits that last longer than is usually the case when a patient is just having a single procedure, such as filling a cavity, performed.

It's important to understand that none of the sedation dentistry techniques, even including IV sedation, involve what's referred to as "deep" or general sedation. Even with IV sedation, the anesthesiologist ordinarily induces a "twilight sedation," one where the patient is under a "light sleep".. They're more in just a state of deep relaxation, sort of between being asleep and somewhat awake.

With the nitrous oxide procedure, which uses the lightest level of sedation, you can usually drive yourself home and resume your normal daily activities within just a few minutes of the time when we turn off the machine used to deliver the sedation. Nitrous oxide procedures typically don't last more than 30 minutes to an hour – in that sense, you can kind of look at it as being similar to novocaine. We prefer to limit using nitrous oxide to no more than an hour because using it any longer than that can cause some patients to begin feeling nauseous.

If you're having oral sedation, you may fall asleep or stay awake, but feel more in that kind of "twilight" level of wakefulness. It varies from person to person. In any case, the sedation, which is deeper than nitrous oxide sedation, but not as deep as the sedation level with IV sedation, wears off more slowly, and that's why we advise you – with either oral or IV sedation - to have someone drive you home, to take the day off from work, and avoid handling any kind of important business dealings, personal or professional. It's a good idea to have a friend or family member stay with you the rest of the day. Usually, by the next day, you should be fine to resume your normal activities.

With IV sedation, you're usually sedated for a few hours. Three to four hours is a general estimate – the time frame might be extended or shortened, just depending on the type of dental work you're having done. Because of our considerable experience, we're pretty good at estimating the time required, and we can get quite a lot of work done within a three to four-hour time frame.

Afterward, you can just go home, sleep for awhile, and a lot of the time, when patients wake up, they don't have any recollection of the dental visit at all. A lot of patients like that, because they don't have any memory of any discomfort at all, and that can help reduce their overall dental anxiety, and make it easier for them to have regular dental work done in the future.

## A LIFE-CHANGING EXPERIENCE

One of the greatest things about sedation dentistry is how it can really impact your life in a hugely positive way. If you've had some significant dental anxiety issues, then sedation dentistry is often the thing that can enable you to finally get that beautiful, healthy smile you've always wanted.

I remember a young man, 26 years old, who was one of our patients who needed a lot of dental work done. He came in with his parents, and it was obvious that he had such a high level of dental anxiety that the only way he would agree to have the work done was if we used the IV sedation. We were able to introduce him to our anesthesiologist here, whom we've known very well for quite some time. Anyway, to make a long story short, using the IV sedation, with four dental professionals including the anesthesiologist and the hygienist, we were able to completely take care of everything that needed to be done in just one visit. And again, this was another case where getting this work done was just a wonderfully life-changing experience for this young man. It changed his whole attitude as far as how he felt about himself and in terms of raising his level of self-esteem and self-confidence – in addition to the fact that he now has just a terrific looking smile. I'm so glad we were able to help him.

Again, dental anxiety is a pretty common condition, so don't be shy about telling your dentist if you do have some anxiety issues. A good dentist realizes that some people have had some bad experiences – like maybe when they had some dental work done when they were a child, the dentist accidentally hit a nerve, causing them to feel sudden pain – that have, quite understandably, left them with some dental anxiety. We respect the fact that your anxiety is a perfectly reasonable and normal way to feel, and we just want to help you deal with it in a way that enables you to take good care of your teeth and your smile.

A lot of times, all it really takes is just coming in for that first visit. If you're anxious about that initial visit, feel free to bring someone along with you, a friend or relative, someone you trust and who can just kind of hold your hand and be there for you. With young people, we often encourage them to bring at least one of their parents along. That's also a good idea because younger people often aren't the ones paying for the treatment, so we want to have the opportunity to explain and discuss the cost issues with their parents if that's who will be paying the bill. But anyway, most of the time if you just come in for that initial consultation, and we have the opportunity to fully explain things to you, including the various options available with sedation dentistry, that alone may reduce a lot of your anxiety, and then you can move forward from there to getting things taken care of.

It's usually helpful just to be able to meet the dental staff at an office beforehand and get to know them and get comfortable with them. During the initial visit, we like to have patients meet our staff, see our offices, and then just talk with us about what you'd like to have done, and what your concerns are. We like to usually try to take care of getting some initial X-rays. That way we can devise a treatment plan to discuss with you and help you decide exactly what you want to get done and how you want it done.

If because of your dental anxiety, you've been putting things off for a long time, and things have gotten to the point where you're in a lot of pain, we, of course, want to address those kinds of immediate, pressing issues in your initial visit. So we're going to do all that we can to make you feel more comfortable as quickly as possible and get the help you need.

Personally, I wish that more patients were made aware of sedation dentistry because I think most people would enjoy more positive dental experiences by taking advantage of the option to have work done with sedation. I know that if I were having a lot of dental work done, I'd certainly choose sedation dentistry.

If you're one of the many people who have dental anxiety issues, try making an appointment to talk with a dentist about sedation dentistry and how it can help you personally in getting a more beautiful, healthy smile.

# ABOUT DR. SHITAL PATEL AND DR. RAKESH PATEL

Dental Care of Corona
DentalCareOfCorona.com

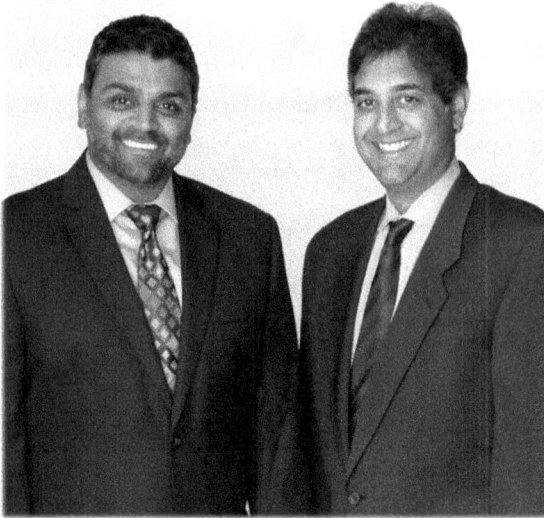

Dr. Shital Patel and Dr. Rakesh Patel of Dental Care of Corona have worked diligently for many years to provide their patients with the very best in professional dental care. With over 25 years of experience each, they firmly believe in providing the highest quality in painless and compassionate care for each individual, whether that means routine preventative dentistry or special services.

Their practice is one of the largest in Corona, CA, offering full service dentistry and orthodontic care. They offer fillings, crowns, periodontal service and implants as well as braces, teeth whitening and many other procedures. Since the practice has a full array of dental specialists, patients do not need to be referred out and can receive comprehensive care under one roof.

Dr. Rakesh Patel graduated from the University of Liverpool in 1992, after which he attended an additional year of training in general dentistry. In 1997, he obtained his license to practice dentistry in California and moved to the United States. Dr. Rakesh Patel serves his patients with compassionate, gentle and expert dental care.

Dr. Shital Patel graduated from the University of Wales in 1991 and continued his training at the University of London for an additional year. He became licensed in California in 1999 and has been practicing with Dr. Rakesh since 2000. Together they serve patients from throughout the Inland Empire and Orange County.

Both Dr. Rakesh and Dr. Shital recognize the importance of staying up to date on all new techniques and technology in order to provide the very best dental care to patients. Both doctors regularly attend continuing education classes to develop these skills and network with other dentists to share ideas.

Dr. Rakesh Patel and Dr. Shital Patel make a difference in people's lives by providing care that exceeds expectations. Along with their competent and friendly staff, these dentists are working to create beautiful smiles that enhance self-esteem and help patients obtain the best possible oral health.

www.ingramcontent.com/pod-product-compliance
Lightning Source LLC
Chambersburg PA
CBHW070909270326
41927CB00011B/2499